LIVE LONGER, HAPPIER & HEALTHIER THROUGH INTERMITTENT FASTING FOR WOMEN OVER 50

All Inclusive Guide for Weight Loss, Exercise Tips and Recipes to Combine With Intermittent Fasting

VIOLET MAY

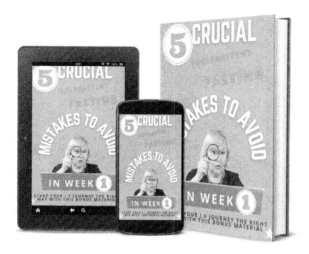

Thank you so much for choosing to read this book. As a gift to my readers I have created an amazing guide to help you make the most of the first week in your intermittent fasting journey. This short guide gives you an overview of the crucial mistakes that are made in week 1 and how you can avoid them. All you need is to scan the QR code at the bottom of the page (use hover over it with the camera open on your phone) click on the link, enter in your email to receive this FREE document, and away you go!

If that doesn't work, please visit violet-may.co.uk and it will take you directly to the page where you can download this guide.

Table of Contents

Introduction

Age is just a number, isn't it? That being said, it's an extremely important and significant number in our lives. It's a number that should be cherished and appreciated. There are so many changes to consider and navigate through this chapter in your life from the joy of grandchildren to the bitter sweet sentiment of retirement. One of the more significant changes around this age is the health of a woman beginning to accelerate towards more unpredictable and sometimes daunting physical changes. There is no magic formula or guide that could literally roll back the years and many claims have been made through books and courses that all promise to be *'the one'*. What this book will not do is give you false claims and guarantees with a route to the fountain of youth. What it will do is give you a tried and tested method successfully used and recommended by millions around the world trying to feel younger, lose stubborn belly fat and gain the energy to live a fulfilling life and not just to get by. Can intermittent fasting really be *'the one'*? This book tailors all the information about intermittent fasting relevant to women in their fifties and beyond. No punches will be pulled, the good, bad and ugly information will be detailed for you to consume about the various methods of intermittent fasting along with recipes and exercise tips to aid you on this exciting journey.

Every one of us has tried a 'diet' at least a handful of times and experimented with a fancy new 'how to look younger' cosmetic fad. The problem is that it always seems to be a temporary fix. You may have seen some results in the form of a few pounds lost but it's never something you can sustain over a prolonged period of time. This normally is because you haven't been given the tools to correctly keep you on track and eventually this will affect your entire mindset towards the goals you want to achieve. The motivation soon turns into despair and BOOM! You're back to square one. The information in this book is underpinned by the failures I and so many have experienced in the journey of weight loss and the learnings of what I needed to do to finally stay on the path towards my goals and not tap out every so often and waste all my hard work. Reading this book will challenge your mindset, help you map out your goals, give you the full scope of intermittent fasting's pros and cons with detail on how to accelerate sustainable weight loss with exercise and recipes.

In America, women have a longer life expectancy than men, and that means they potentially have a longer period of developing health problems as they grow older. So, while you celebrate your 50's and beyond, you should also be aware of some of the health related hurdles you are more susceptible to and know how to give yourself the best chance to navigate over them *(don't worry, no actual hurdling is required of you in any of the intermittent fasting plans!)* It may come as no surprise to know, your body is as aware of the stage of life you are entering into even more so than your family and friends that may have spent months preparing that big 50th or 60th party. If you haven't prepared your body and health for this new stage in your life, it's not too late to make a radical, safe and transformational change through this book's guidance on intermittent fasting.

Intermittent fasting as a concept is extremely simple, flexible and adaptable to any lifestyle. In Layman's terms, you will be setting a schedule for the week in which every day you will have a period of time you have no food and a period shortly after that where you can eat food. Simple right? A key study done in 2019 simplified intermittent fasting down to; *'involving you modifying your eating schedule and breaking it into a period of eating and fasting'*. There are about four well known eating schedules in intermittent fasting, and they have different eating plans. In this book, you will get to know about the different eating schedules and how they work; then, you can decide which one will work best for you.

The traditional thinking that intermittent fasting is a way of starving yourself couldn't be further from the truth. The reality is, according to multiple articles, our bodies can go for weeks without food before we actually start 'starving'. Is this an endorsement to abstain from food for that long, absolutely not! The point is to illustrate that despite how we might feel when we don't eat food, our bodies are more than capable of adapting, even in extreme scenarios of not consuming any food for weeks. With intermittent fasting, there is a requirement to abstain from food, unfortunately there is no way around it. The reasoning behind why is not down to punishing your body, it is essentially to create a calorie deficit. In some plans it could be 24 hours of no eating and in others it may only be ⅓ of the day- with both options potentially being as successful as each other depending on various factors such as what food you eat in your feasting window- more to come on this later. This should give you the confidence that despite the hunger pains you might feel, your body will adapt and thrive. Will your body like it at first- no! Will your body begin to accept and get used to what you tell it to do- yes! One of the main reasons why the health of an aging body begins to deteriorate outside of biology and the natural decline we can all expect, is we are so used to our bodies dictating what and when we eat. So many of us are governed by the *want* of our body as opposed to the *need* and the two are easily confused. Many times, if we have a bad day for example, our body tells us we *need* to overindulge with food and beverages that our body doesn't actually need and in the end we actually don't feel any better. There is a control that most have lost over their body and the results of this lack of discipline and control is evident through health decline, weight issues and so many other areas of our lives. Intermittent fasting is a tool that will bring structure and ultimately help you take back the control of your body and end the cycle of control your body has over you.

With a structured plan for a new eating schedule, you will take back control of the direction of your body shape, health and where your mental wellbeing is heading in. Your body will resist this change because it is used to dictating what you eat, when you eat and how you eat. Like a spoiled child our bodies have had no discipline or structure for years. At the very first implementation of this structured eating schedule, our body may kick and scream, cry and stomp its proverbial feet because it is not getting what it 'thinks' you need and is not in control anymore- you are, you will be, through intermittent fasting.

Beyond losing weight and staying in shape, intermittent fasting has more benefits than you can imagine. While you may only be considering its weight loss benefits, intermittent fasting provides other health benefits for your physical and mental health. Intermittent fasting helps to improve your muscle and joint health, depression, lowers your risk of diseases like heart diseases, cancer, diabetes, metabolic diseases, reduces your blood sugar and insulin levels.

Our bodies are smart, flexible and most importantly different. Each person's biological make-up is unique and requires different approaches when it comes to effective weight loss or health improvement techniques. This is why most diets work for the first few weeks, then your body adapts and your results plateau. This book will walk you through an array of different exercise techniques to combine with your intermittent fasting to keep your body in sync with your desired destination. We will also explore various recipes that specifically target areas of your health that you want to improve such as, skin care, brain health, increasing your energy and so much more. Is this style of weight loss suitable for most people? Absolutely. There are however some exceptions to this through pre-existing health conditions, medication and other elements, but this will all be explored and explained in beginning chapters. Through the guidance of this book you will be able to choose from a multitude of recipes and various intermittent fasting plans to mould and shape to fit your desired outcome.

Enjoyment doesn't have to stop at fifty, be it on your taste buds or body. You can still enjoy delicious healthy meals and look as young as you desire. Do you want to make intermittent fasting a lifestyle while you rock your fifties in style? Do you want to know how you can do this? Proceed to read the rest of the book. Enjoy!

Chapter One:

How Your Body and Intermittent Fasting Can Work Together

Years ago I used to work in a business looking after accounts for a local van rental company. The money was really good and most of my colleagues were around my age and had similar interests. Most weekends there was a work party to go to and of course, I would be the first person there and probably the last to leave. Spur of the moment weekends away, guilt free shopping every month and no real concern financially; i have the money, why not spend it? I ended up working at this company for a long period of time and became really close with a lot of great people. One of those people was a girl named Hayley. Although we were close, she very rarely joined us on night outs and these expensive trips we used to make and at first I thought nothing of it but after a while it became really noticeable. She was prudent with her finances and not as carefree as the rest of us. A few years had gone by and one morning I was in the office kitchen and she came bursting through the doors. Hayley came in screaming 'I DID IT!' After just about saving the coffee in my cup from spilling onto my hands through the shock of her entrance, I calmed her down and asked her to explain what she actually did. It turns out, Hayley had bought her first house. For the past 5 years she had been saving every month in anticipation of this day. All the times she had declined certain events or holidays away, she was putting money aside for her future. She was extremely happy but also visibly emotional because of all the sacrifices she had made to set up her future. What has this got to do with intermittent fasting? The truth is, the way we treat our health is similar to my lifestyle at this workplace. We tend not to see any tangible consequences to being carefree with what we eat or how we treat our bodies when we were younger so we don't invest in our futures through some sacrifice right now. Through many years of bad eating habits and lack of concern for our health parallel to our decline in age, we are building a biological debt that must be paid. The evidence of this 'payment' is seen in various ways that manifest through high blood pressure, unhealthy skin, sustained weight gain, weak bones and so many other facets.

As we get older our body begins to fail us. Some of it is down to Mother Nature, however a lot of the ailments women over 50 suffer with are down to years of over indulging and a lack of sacrifice for your body's benefit in the future. It may not be as drastic as your body literally breaking down. Some women just don't like the way they look anymore. That feeling of your youth being a distant memory and the 'biological debt' is what you see in the mirror instead of the woman you want to be. This by no means is a path that cannot be reversed and you are in the right place because intermittent fasting is an amazing tool to help you do just that.

With the major development in medicine and healthcare the human race is able to live longer. Diseases that would shorten our life expectancy a few decades ago are still dangerous now, but through highly developed medicine, the average age of the population across the country is increasing. At face value, this sounds like a safety blanket for us all- medicine. The reality is, who wants to rely on being medicated, hospitalised or under the supervision of a nurse if they could potentially avoid it? Sometimes this may be unavoidable and that's where medical care is so vital, however our lifestyle and food choices contribute towards a lot of ailments and diseases that women over 50 become more prone to. Taking this into account, is intermittent fasting a replacement for our healthcare and medical recommendations? No. It is, however, a natural method of enhancing our bodies' resilience against some of the most debilitating diseases known to us today. Intermittent fasting is a means of giving our bodies the best chance of preventing our health getting into a position whereby being medicated becomes part of our lives and not an occasional addition. As the saying goes, prevention is better than cure. This chapter will educate you on the likely changes you are going to experience and how intermittent fasting can help your body during these changes. That being said, the aging body is not a prerequisite to ailments and not everyone experiences major deterioration as they grow older. Mother Nature has taught us that we are more *likely* to experience these biological challenges when we are over 50 and the next portion of the book is to give you an overview of the possible ailments that you may experience that intermittent fasting can help negate.

Understanding Your Body at 50+

Whether you are generally healthy and just looking to shave a few pounds or your health seems to be a constant issue, understanding potential health related hurdles as you enter this new chapter of life is important. Similar to a teenager experiencing the early stages of puberty, these changes to the body can be daunting. Your body is still a wonderfully complex design that may be showing new signs of unwanted changes. The list we will go through is certainly not a predetermined destination for women over 50. It is however important to understand some of the health related obstacles women who reach this amazing milestone may experience. Remember, all of the changes we will go through can be slowed down, brought under control or sometimes completely eradicated through intermittent fasting.

Weight gain and belly fat

Many people dread weight gain, especially when it is unhealthy and drastic. Simple things like not fitting into your favorite dresses or jeans anymore can be extremely disheartening! It also means that you have more work to do if you want to shed the unwanted fat. Who doesn't want to enjoy their plates of goodies anytime they want? Who doesn't want to have to never hit the gym? You want to eat anything you desire without worrying about gaining weight. But for anyone over 50, you may need to consider your health more than you ever did.

The Center for Disease Control and Prevention says that men and women gain at least one to two pounds yearly between early adulthood and middle age. So, weight gain is prevalent among adults above 50. Women especially gain belly fat as soon as they hit menopause. This, however, doesn't mean that menopause directly causes weight gain or belly fat in women. Menopause directly influences hormonal changes in women and it is these hormonal changes that can cause you to gain weight or belly fat.

Also, your body becomes more resistant to insulin as you age. This results in you gaining weight specifically around the belly. When your body becomes resistant to insulin, your fat, muscles, and liver cells don't respond to insulin. So, consequently, your liver cells won't absorb glucose from your bloodstream, resulting in high blood sugar levels. These high blood sugar levels then could result in type 2 diabetes. These chain of events do not occur overnight. The resistance to insulin does not apply to every single woman who is getting older and this may seem extreme. For some women however, this can become a reality and through some positive lifestyle decisions one small step at a time, you can reduce the chances of these detrimental changes in your health.

Metabolism changes

As you age, you begin to experience metabolism changes. These metabolic changes result in weight gain. Your metabolism begins to drop from around your early thirties and will continue dropping as you age. When your metabolism reduces, it is easier for you to add more pounds and it becomes even harder to lose those pounds. Your metabolism burns down your calories, but once it slows down, the number of calories you burn daily reduces as well, resulting in you adding weight. As you age, your activity and productivity reduce, and this contributes to reduced metabolism. The aging of your internal components and muscle loss also reduces your metabolism.

Muscle loss

Muscle loss also relates to weaker bones and can lead or contribute to osteoporosis. A study by AARP found out that 73% of their 1,500 person's survey confirms that they lost muscle as they age, and 13% of the study population knew the importance of maintaining their muscle as they age. The survey also revealed that some of the respondents were hospitalized after 50 due to some chronic diseases, muscle loss, and strength loss.

A recent study done by The Journal of Neurological Sciences found that most women will experience muscle loss of up to 40% by the time they get to 80. This is a sobering thought! The loss of muscle tends to be gradual from our 30's and begins to accelerate as we get closer to our 60's. The term for this gradual muscle loss is sarcopenia. Simultaneously the body of a woman is becoming more susceptible to weight gain and so that leaves us with a troubling combination of muscle loss and weight gain naturally occurring simultaneously. The domino effect of this gradual decline in muscle and increase in weight gain results in loss of strength, more stress on your bones and frailty.

Reduced collagen production

Everyone wants their skin to be radiant and beautiful all the time. Unfortunately, it is not something everyone gets to enjoy due to different reasons. Aging can also prevent you from having glowing, radiant skin, and this can happen due to reduced collagen production. What is collagen, and what does it do to your skin?

Collagen is a protein that helps keep your skin firm and elastic. A generous amount of collagen in your skin is why you enjoyed beautiful, radiant skin when you were younger. The production of collagen reduces as you age and your skin might get wrinkled. This is a huge reason why the cosmetic industry has made billions of dollars through medically reducing this symptom of ageing. Fortune Business evaluated the Botox industry in 2019 and found the industry to be worth just over $4 billion and projected to be worth in excess of £7 billion by 2027. Whether this appetite to reduce wrinkles is down to how the media have created an insecurity for 'looking old' or not, there is clearly a fear of showing signs of ageing. There are elements of intermittent fasting with tailored recipes that could boost collagen and certainly make improvements with your skin's appearance and if you want a more natural way of doing this, you're in the right place! There are much more natural and sustainable ways of boosting collagen through food choices and lifestyle both of which intermittent fasting will propel you towards.

Hormonal effects and menopause

Women start experiencing menopause when they are around age 50. This means that your ovaries begin to produce a lesser amount of estrogen, progesterone and a large amount of follicle-stimulating hormone (FSH). When women go through menopause, they experience different side effects, and they vary in different individuals. When you are going through menopause, you are likely to experience insomnia, mood swings, hot flushes, decreased sex drive and sometimes either mild or aggressive symptoms of depression.

I know what you're thinking, growing old sucks! All of these ailments and problems are just waiting in my biological path. That doesn't have to be the case at all. Many women get older and do not entertain intermittent fasting, exercise or healthy meal plans and never experience any major health setbacks. It is, however, a bit of a biological lottery. Some are lucky enough to not have to consider their lifestyle choices and not hit many health related bumps in the road. For many others, that simply just is not the case.

The data however tells us that due to the types of food that we are all exposed to don't give you the best chance of not experiencing any major health setbacks. Fast food and highly concentrated sugar snacks are so good and much more attractive than healthy options. Busy lifestyles with work, social events and family can be consuming. The truth is, most women's health is taking a back seat to other priorities. Because most don't see the harm of neglecting a healthy lifestyle with immediate consequences, life just continues as normal. The body's natural biological trajectory is downward and this is accelerated by lifestyle choices. As our age increases, our bodies begin to show the effects of slowly breaking down and this is what may open the door to some health related complications. But it's never too late to affect that trajectory. Through the rest of this chapter you will begin to understand the benefits of how intermittent fasting can be a huge step in the direction of repairing your body internally and seeing those results manifest through weight loss, mental wellbeing and so much more!

What is Intermittent Fasting, and How Does it Help You?

At this point, there is a need to clarify that intermittent fasting isn't a diet. It is more like you deciding when to eat and when to stay away from food. It is a pattern of eating. The attractiveness of intermittent fasting tends to be around the notion that you can eat whatever you want during your feasting window. To a degree, this is true. The theory behind this statement is that if you limit your eating to a smaller window in your 24 hrs, you're likely to consume less calories than if you had the whole day to freely consume food. A well respected commentator in the intermittent fasting space Kristin Koskinen, RDN states that *'technically, there are no diet restrictions with intermittent fasting, it's an eating style that is based on food timing rather than diet composition'*. That being said, making subtle changes to what you eat can accelerate the effects that intermittent fasting has on weight loss specifically. As mentioned previously, there is not one person on earth who can claim to have never been an undisciplined eater. We have all over indulged, over-eaten and had one or two (maybe 10) too many glasses of wine. Ultimately, the effectiveness of intermittent fasting comes down to creating a calorie deficit. Every day you are burning calories whether you know it or not and an article in The Healthline describes the three ways you are doing so as the following;

- **Resting energy expenditure (REE):** REE refers to the calories your body uses at rest for functions that maintain your body's functions, such as breathing and blood circulation.

- **Thermic effect of food:** This involves the calories your body expends digesting, absorbing, and metabolizing food.

- **Activity energy expenditure:** Calories you burn during exercise and other non-exercise related activities that require you to exert energy such as household cleaning.

In order to create this deficit you need to know what your 'maintenance calories' are. Maintenance calories are the amount of calories your body needs in order to support your daily expenditure of energy and generally for a woman over 50 the maintenance calorie number is around 1,800 calories per day. This will vary depending on age, current weight, height and physical activity. Once you know this number, if you consume anything less than your maintenance number every day, let's say 1,400 calories, you are creating a calorie deficit of 400 calories. This in turn will trigger your body to burn stored fat thus creating weight loss. There are many ways to find out your exact maintenance number and creating that deficit might mean you need to know exactly how many calories you are eating each day. The thought of 'calorie counting' to many is arduous and over complicated and understandably so. You do not have to necessarily count your calories to create a deficit. Although the creation of apps, required calorie information displayed on food, BMI calculators and many other resources are available to accurately determine these numbers, although really useful, it's not absolutely necessary to make this work. Later on in the book you will find some useful guides on how to take measurements and apps to assist in really elevating you towards your goals. As you begin, if you work on the premise of replacing some of the really unhealthy food you consume with some wholesome nutritious food all within your feasting window, you will no doubt create a deficit just on that basis. If you find that the weight loss is not progressing as quickly as you like, all you need to do is either increase your activity or change your diet slightly. Make the small steps first before you worry about some of the more complicated elements of calorie counting! Although this deficit is important in creating weight loss, it is not the entire story as calories are not the only thing to affect weight. More to come on this later in the book.

Below is a useful chart to give you an idea of what your maintenance calories would roughly be based on age, being female and how active you are. Any calories consumed below this number, is a great start to losing weight.

Females

Age	Inactive	Moderate	Active
51–60	1,600	1,800	2,200
61+	1,600	1,800	2,000

Benefits of Intermittent Fasting

You should look beyond the weight loss benefits of intermittent fasting and at other ways IF can be beneficial to you. IF is beneficial to women's health in many ways, like the following:

Cancer

Cancer is one of the most diagnosed diseases among women, and about 8.2 million deaths in 2012 were cancer-related and that number has increased exponentially since. Women battle different cancers, ranging from breast, cervix, lung, stomach, colorectal cancers. Out of all of these, breast cancer is the second most diagnosed form of cancer that women experience. Intermittent fasting, however, is a tool that research has pointed towards potentially helping fight the causes of cancer and aid in the process of recovery from cancer. It can potentially help slow down the progression of cancer as studies have shown that fasting improves insulin sensitivity. This essentially means that cells can metabolize insulin more efficiently aiding the removal of glucose from the blood. Intermittent fasting also boosts your immune system. Researchers have found that intermittent fasting can also help cancer treatments like chemotherapy and radiotherapy be more effective by attacking cancer malignancies in the body and enabling cancer cells to be more responsive to treatment (Nair and Khawale, 2016).

Musculoskeletal health

Your musculoskeletal health is important, and health conditions that relate to it can have serious effects on your life. These conditions can lead to serious long-term pain, physical disability, and it affects a large number of people in the world. These conditions can either be short-term or be life-long conditions like arthritis, osteoporosis, back pain, etc. As we all age, we are at more risk of having these conditions and many have found intermittent fasting to be an amazing deterrent to these potential ailments.

Intermittent fasting affects parathyroid hormone secretion, which is good for your body. Intermittent fasting impacts your circadian rhythm. When your circadian rhythm is altered, it affects your parathyroid hormone, which results in calcium, phosphate metabolism and bone remodeling. Intermittent fasting helps to reduce inflammation and its mediators, like, cytokines, leukotrienes, and prostaglandins. A study revealed that fasting between 7 to 10 days helped reduce pain, stiffness, and dependency on analgesics in RA patients. Inflammation is a contributing factor to musculoskeletal disorders and intermittent fasting helps reduce it.

As you age, you are likely to have osteoporosis and other illnesses related to fractures, this has been a source of concern for many people. As people grow older, there has been a high mortality rate from fractures as a result of low bone density minerals. Calorie reduction and fasting can help slow down the growth of age-related diseases. Other findings also show that fasting can help reduce your body weight and body mass, resulting in the reduction of risks of adults having fractures and other comorbidities.

Metabolic health

When you are 50 and above, your metabolism level drops, as you have read before. That makes you prone to some metabolism abnormalities, like, increased abdominal fat, reduced high-density lipoprotein, increased glucose and insulin levels, etc. Intermittent fasting can, however, help improve your metabolic health. IF helps you with weight loss, reduction in blood pressure, fat tissue mass, heart rate, etc. It also helps you with improving your lipid profile, HDL cholesterol level and decreases your total cholesterol and LDL cholesterol level (Anson, Guo, de Cabo, Iyun, Rios, Hagepanos, Ingram, Lane, and Mattson, 2003).

Intermittent fasting will help reduce the weight in your waist area, and at the same time, improve your insulin sensitivity. That is to say, intermittent fasting can help improve the metabolic dysfunction you are already experiencing or might experience in the future.

Mental health

One reason women go through mental health difficulties can be due to hormonal changes, especially when entering into or going through menopause. Studies show 80-85% of women experience menopausal symptoms at different points of their menopausal transition. When you are going through menopause, you are likely to experience moodiness, tension, hot flashes, anxiety and emotional instability. The *Journal of Nutrition Health & Aging* did a study and found that after three months of fasting, participants reported an improved mood, reduced anxiety, lowered tension and decreased feelings of anger. Part of this is due to the fact that intermittent fasting triggers autophagy. This is the process of the brain essentially clearing out old and damaged cells and promoting the regeneration of new healthy cells.

This cleansing of the body's old cells is like the mental trash is being taken out and replaced with new furniture, a scented candle and soft relaxing music. That might not be everyone's ideal replacement for trash so feel free to imagine whatever replacement you like! The point being, your mood and mental health is linked to your chemical makeup neurologically and intermittent fasting has a positive impact on this.

When You Should Avoid Intermittent Fasting

The benefits of intermittent fasting are widely experienced by beginners and those that have adopted this as a lifestyle over a prolonged period of time. Although this is true, this method is not suitable for everyone. There are some instances where intermittent fasting should be avoided as it could potentially do more harm than good. Some people might experience serious side effects, and that is why some healthcare professionals advise some individuals not to practice intermittent fasting.

So, who shouldn't practice intermittent fasting? Intermittent fasting isn't for:

- Women who are breastfeeding or pregnant.
- Young children and teenagers
- Older adults who experience weakness in their body
- People with dementia
- People with eating disorders, whether past or present
- People with immunodeficiencies
- People who have had a traumatic brain injury or post-concussive syndrome in the past

Apart from these, if you have a medical condition and you are currently taking medication, you should ask your doctor or healthcare provider if it is safe for you to practice intermittent fasting. You don't want to risk experiencing any complications or side effects that do more harm than good, so it's safer that you consult your doctor. It will do no harm to your journey by consulting medical guidance from your doctor prior to taking on intermittent fasting. This journey may be such a big step change for your body that getting your bloods done, having a conversation with your doctor, someone who understands your medical history could be hugely beneficial in giving you some understanding as your body begins to adapt.

Intermittent fasting's side effects include extreme hunger, nausea, faintness, headaches, fatigue, irritability. So, if you are experiencing really terrible side effects, you should stop immediately. There is a big difference between feeling hungry and slightly irritable which is normal when you first start fasting compared to some of the more extreme side effects mentioned earlier. This is why it is key for some consultation with a medical professional to help recognise the difference between your body telling you to stop because you are causing harm and your mind telling you to stop because change is daunting. As I said at the beginning of the book, I want this book to give you the full scope of this eating schedule, the good, bad and ugly! Intermittent fasting might not work for everyone, and its okay if it doesn't work for you.

That being said, there are many discussions about how intermittent fasting works and a lot of 'myths' circulating around this topic. I refer to them as myths because there are a lot of misconceptions about IF (intermittent fasting) that either are not scientifically backed and some that are just flat out untrue. The rest of this chapter will detail some of the common myths surrounding intermittent fasting and if you should take them into consideration during your pursuit of health and wellbeing.

Myths about Intermittent Fasting

Skipping breakfast leads to promoting weight gain

One you may have heard is that you will experience serious hunger if you skip meals, which leads to cravings and then weight gain. A 16-week study showed that the respondents who skipped breakfast and those who didn't skip breakfast didn't experience any weight difference.

So, if you have been scared that you might gain weight instead of losing it if you skip a meal, you are wrong. Breakfast doesn't really affect your weight, whether you skip it or not. Although breakfast is good for you to perform better during the day, skipping it might not do you any harm. However, you should pay attention to your body's needs, so you can know whether it is good for you or not. Keep in mind, the IF plans are flexible and you can incorporate the plans to accommodate your lifestyle. If you find that skipping breakfast does not work for you, adjust the plan to make sure you have breakfast and sacrifice other meals later in the day. Once you get to the section detailing the plans, it will all make more sense.

Frequent eating boosts your metabolism

Another common thought is that the more you eat, the higher your metabolic rate, which equates to you burning more calories. The truth is, your body burns some calories when digesting food through a process known as the thermic effect of food (TEF). TEF burns 10% of the calories you consume on average. So, what actually matters is not the number of times you eat or the quantity. What matters is the number of calories you consume. So, you burn an average of 10% of calories in all the meals you eat. Increasing or reducing how much you eat doesn't increase or decrease the usual calories your body burns during digestion.

Frequent eating helps reduce hunger

You have probably heard that you can prevent yourself from having cravings or feeling excessive hunger if you eat frequently. Research concerning this claim is conflicting. Some studies found it to be true, while others found it not to be true. Whether frequent eating helps reduce hunger or not depends on the individuals. There is no proof that frequent eating or snacking can reduce hunger.

Frequently eating is good for your health

People have probably told you that eating often is good for your health. It is quite the opposite. When you are without food, your body starts a process mentioned earlier called autophagy, in which the body repairs your cells, and your cell uses old and dysfunctional proteins for energy.

Autophagy is widely recognised as a deterrent for Alzheimer's disease. Fasting is also good for your metabolic health. Eating frequently, especially unhealthy meals, can pose more harm to your health than good. A particular study found out that frequently eating high calorie meals can increase your liver fat and your risk of having fatty liver which can lead to health difficulties.

Fasting puts your body in starvation mode

A common belief that people have about fasting is that it puts you in starvation mode, thereby slowing down metabolism and hinders you from burning your body fat. It is true that long-term weight loss can reduce the number of calories you burn over time; however, this happens irrespective of the fasting or a weight loss process you choose.

A short-term fast can increase your metabolic rate because the blood levels of your norepinephrine increase drastically, and it triggers your metabolism and your fat cells to break down your body fats. Studies have shown that 48 hours of fasting can increase your metabolism by up to 3.6% to 14%. Therefore, fasting does not put your body into starvation mode as mentioned in the introduction, starvation occurs after a sustained period of weeks of not eating anything at all.

Your body only uses a certain amount of protein in every meal you eat

Some people believe that you can only digest 30 grams of protein per meal, so you need to eat every two to three hours to get more protein and maximize muscle gain. But this isn't backed by science, so it might not be true. However, a study showed that eating protein in frequent food servings doesn't affect your muscle mass. The important thing you should be concerned about is ensuring that you eat the required amount of protein your body needs instead of eating a large amount in different servings or in a single serving.

Intermittent fasting makes you overeat

Another misconception is that fasting leads to cravings which makes you overeat during the eating period. It is true that after fasting, you might want to compensate by overeating a little bit, but that isn't all that is there to it. A particular study showed that the respondents who fasted for 24 hours ended up eating about 1,400 calories the next day, but this is less compared to the 2,400 calories they would've consumed if they weren't fasting.

So, intermittent fasting doesn't make you gain weight but helps you lose it. It may feel like you are overeating during your eating period, but you are also reducing the calorie and junk you were likely to eat for the whole day if you weren't fasting.

Intermittent fasting works for everyone

Although the benefits are huge and many have raved about the results, the research related to this topic is somewhat limited in comparison to other weight loss techniques or methods. Do not be disheartened if this method does not work for you, IF is not a universal guarantee for weight loss and health improvement. The simplified deduction of IF is essentially being mindful of what you are eating and being aware of your biological makeup to enhance the results. This is set out in a framework of plans or schedules to create a structure to follow (16:8, 5:2 – more detail on these plans later this chapter). For some, this structure is useful, for others not so much. The key here is to understand that the benefits are amazing, but do not feel like if it doesn't work for you, there is no other way to achieve the results you need.

You can eat whatever you want in your feasting window

This train of thought is underpinned by what has been relayed earlier in the book. Generally, when there are no constraints we tend to eat way more calories because we are subject to 'mindless eating'. IF introduces 'mindful eating' where we are more considered and restricted by an eating window. This may mean we are likely to eat less because we have a smaller window to do so, therefore eating whatever you like is not a problem. The problem with this train of thought is you may eat less calories, but if you do not make a slight adaptation on the types of foods you consume, you will slow down your progress.

At 50, you have probably been hearing people advising you about how important it is to take care of your health. Being 50 doesn't mean you lose your glow or your agility, but it does mean that you are entering a period where you have to be careful about your health. You are likely to gain weight, lose muscle, experience hormonal changes, metabolic changes and you need a plan to help you scale through those periods and live healthily for many years to come. One way you can stay healthy and in shape is through intermittent fasting. With IF, you can lose weight, reduce your risks of having some diseases and you can live a longer and healthy life. There are also some myths you have probably heard that may be discouraging you from trying intermittent fasting and they have been explored with some context in this chapter. So, you have all the information you need to make an informed decision. You should also know that intermittent fasting isn't for everyone, so you should consult your doctor before you start, especially if you are on any medication. Also, if you are experiencing serious side effects while you are fasting, you might want to stop fasting and consider other health orientated methods to reach your goals.

You have more exciting things to learn in this book, including recipes you can try out. But, there is no rush, one step at a time. So, in the next chapter, you will get to know about the different types of intermittent fasting, their pros and cons, and how you can pick the right one. There are options you can pick from for your fasting practice, so get ready to be enlightened.

Chapter Two:

The Pros and Cons for Types of Intermittent Fasting

Just as it's fit for you to know what intermittent fasting is all about, it is equally important you know that there are different approaches to this eating plan. There are some methods that require a lot of sacrifice and there are other methods that you can adjust to fit around your lifestyle. This chapter will explore all of the most popular forms of IF and give you a breakdown of the pros and cons of each method. The key considerations to make (which will be explored later in the book) are your goals and your lifestyle commitments. Remember, the goal of IF is to give you a structure to your eating habits. Start with a plan that is easy to adopt and gradually build to more difficult structures to give yourself the best chance of seeing the amazing results so many participants have seen.

Many women above fifty make a common mistake when they are considering weight loss and that is choosing an intermittent fasting method without consulting their doctor. So, they choose without taking time to understand the principles of each of the plans. The point is that, although they likely produce the same result, their regulations differ.

At your wonderful age, weight loss doesn't come as easy as you might have thought. One of the main reasons is due to the decreased metabolism many face as they get older. The process of digestion takes more time than usual when you reach your fifties. You know why? The enzymes that are responsible for breaking down food in different organs become weaker. There are so many things accountable for that as well. Where this has manifested itself is through late night snacking or meals that are consumed close to the time you go to bed. That action has caused more harm than good for the enzymes aiding metabolism. Some have problems with their genetic make-up. These, among others, are responsible for such reactions. However, we have lean muscle that makes metabolism faster and easier when we are younger. But as soon as we start to approach 50, we begin to lose muscle mass. And as a result of that, we become less active than when we were younger.

Research has shown that intermittent fasting has a lot of benefits. Part of it is that it would help to improve your metabolism. Intermittent fasting is pretty advantageous, but it is helpful to know what types of demands and purpose they are made to achieve. But before adopting it, consider a few things.

The fact that none of these types of intermittent fasting are one size fits all, especially for those approaching 50 and beyond, is an enough reason why you should take your time to know the type that's the best fit for you.

That's why in choosing a plan type, you have to consider your goal alongside your age. The body becomes susceptible and reacts so quickly to anything we eat or the things we do. That's why it is important to know the pros and cons of each of the types of intermittent fasting to be sure of the result you would get after engaging in it.

Such knowledge would not only help you choose wisely; it would also help you to make an informed decision about your health. Although numerous essentials are accrued to intermittent fasting, the misuse or abuse of it might cause side effects that would water down the goals it is meant to achieve. That being said, let's explore!

Types of Intermittent Fasting

Like you have read, there are different types of intermittent fasting. The methods vary in the number of days and the calorie intake. Skipping food for some days or times and the number of calories allowed makes these methods differ from one another. Once you understand these differences; you would be able to make a choice that ultimately will get you to your goals. Below are the popular types with their strengths and weaknesses. You should read and choose the best plan fit for you. But remember, you need to involve your doctor.

The 16:8 Method

This method of IF is suggested for beginners because it is extremely flexible and you can change the ratio between your eating and non-eating period according to whichever time frame fits around your lifestyle best and degree of difficulty you want to implement. 16:8 is the ratio of hours between fasting and non fasting periods in a 24 hour timeframe. You can scale up and scale down the ratio as you become more confident and comfortable with this style of IF. There is however a recommended period of time within the day that this plan works the best due to how our body's work. This type of dietary plan reduces the eating period to eight-hours. Between the hours of 9 am to 5 pm, or 11 am to 7 pm. This diet restriction is aimed at boosting the metabolism by introducing fasting for the burning of fats period. Your eating window can end around early evening because it is at this time that metabolism slows down. It is advisable that your fasting window include the hours you spend sleeping. It is also massively beneficial that you don't eat any food two to three hours before you sleep. This will allow your digestive system not to be overworked while you sleep because it has to break down food while you sleep and are inactive, increasing the chances of fat being stored. Remember, if you have a work schedule that doesn't allow you to implement the plan at traditional times best associated with a 9-5 job, do not be afraid to adjust the plan according to your lifestyle. The beauty of this is that you can tweak the plan as necessary as you like to find the sweet spot for you and your goals.

How to do this

16/8 intermittent fasting is simple and easy.

You can start by picking an eight-hour window and limit your food intake to that time span.

Most people prefer eating between noon and 8 pm, as this means you'll only need to fast overnight and skip breakfast but can still eat a balanced lunch and dinner, along with a few healthy snacks throughout the day.

Others may eat between 9 a.m. and 5 p.m, which allows plenty of time for a healthy breakfast around 9 am, a normal lunch around noon and a light early dinner or snack around 4 p.m. before starting your fast. You may also want to consider having a more flexible approach on the weekend when you first begin allowing yourself sometime over the weekend to not be as restrictive. Giving your body a reprieve over the weekend will help keep your metabolism on its toes so to speak and not allow your body to get too used to the routine resulting in a weight loss plateau. You also want to give yourself the chance to enjoy a glass of wine or meal with friends on the weekend without worrying about a fasting window. The last thing you want is to burn out or despise the plan you have because it's restricting your social life too much. It's a balance you must find. That being said you could also go the full seven days committed to your plan and see what the results are after a couple of weeks. The point is to try and test different routines and see what best fits your lifestyle and goals.

An example of an 8 hours eating window could be between:

- 9 am to 5 pm
- 10 am to 6 pm
- 12 pm to 8 pm

Example of the 12 pm-8 pm schedule;

Fasting or Eating	Fasting Period 9 am - 12 pm	Eating Period 12 pm - 8 pm	Fasting Period 8 pm - 9 am
Monday	Fast	Eat	Fast
Tuesday	Fast	Eat	Fast
Wednesday	Fast	Eat	Fast
Thursday	Fast	Eat	Fast
Friday	Fast	Eat	Fast
Saturday	Flexible	Flexible	Flexible
Sunday	Flexible	Flexible	Flexible

If your goal is to burn fat or rev up your metabolism, this kind of fasting is the best fit for you. Let's proceed to study both the pros and cons of this type of intermittent fasting.

Pros

1. Planning meals

Knowing there is an 8 hour window you will be able to eat within should encourage you to plan your meals ahead of time. Planning healthy meals will help you to be mindful of what you're eating and massively benefit your pursuit for health and weight loss.

2. Late night eating

Late night meals are the downfall of many. This plan eliminates late night eating which helps promote a healthier digestive system resulting in huge health benefits.

3. Flexibility

Participants can mould and shape this plan to fit their lifestyles and it is really easy to make the necessary changes when you need to scale the ratio of fasting/non-fasting up or down depending on your lifestyle.

Cons

1. Eat whatever you like

Although planning your meals should encourage you to eat healthier, this requires discipline to do. This plan allows you to eat whatever you like in your eating phase which may result in overeating. Remember, it doesn't have to be this way. The 'eat whatever you like' motto associated with IF can be a counterproductive attitude if it is not monitored.

2. Calories In vs Calories Out

This goes hand in hand with the point above. You are restricting your eating to a period of time in a day therefore the expectation is that you are likely to eat less calories than you would on a normal day because of the time constraint. This however, may not be the case. If you over indulge in your eating phase, you may overcompensate and there may not be any calorie reduction on your fasting days. This would be counterintuitive to the goals you're trying to achieve. The way to negate this is to be mindful of what you eat! Also, being aware of your maintenance weight (discussed earlier) would be useful in having a reference point to stay under and avoid going overboard.

3. Longevity

The success of any weight loss endeavour centres around discipline. This method of IF is dictated by a high level of discipline in meal planning and being mindful of what you are eating. The continuous need for this may result in some losing the motivation to maintain this long term.

5:2 Intermittent Fasting method

Another type of intermittent fasting is known as the Fast Diet. It involves reducing eating habits for two days of the week. It is a type of dietary plan that allows you to normally eat for five days of the week and restrict calories for two days.

This fasting method is good for women above fifty who are trying to lose weight quickly and improve their health status. If you engage in this method of intermittent fasting, you tend to limit calories to about 500-600 daily on the days of your fast.

While you are on this dietary plan, you can normally eat for five days. Eating normal foods implies you can eat to get the average calories that you need within that period of five days. However, that doesn't mean you should overeat during your non-fasting days. This method is also normally branded with 'eat whatever you like when you are not fasting'. The thinking behind this plan is that you are due to restrict your calories on two days and therefore if you eat like you normally would over the other 5, you will see a calorie reduction in your week and therefore lose weight.

How to do this

There are three schedules you can choose from for the 5:2 diet plan. They are:

- You can restrict calories on Monday and Thursday in a week.

- You can also restrict calories on Tuesday and Thursday and eat normally for the remaining days of the week.

- Friday and Sunday are the other days you can restrict your calorie intake.

Days	Food to eat
Monday	500 Calories
Tuesday	Normal food with calories

Wednesday	Normal food with calories
Thursday	500 Calories
Friday	Normal food with calories
Saturday	Normal food with calories
Sunday	Normal food with calories

Pros

1. Make it your own

Have plans on Saturday? Change your fasting day to Monday. This plan is one you can make your own and choose your own fasting days based on your plans every week.

2. Longevity

Due to the flexible nature of this plan on a week to week basis, it is much easier to adapt into your long term plans.

3. Suitable for beginners

You would only be restricting your calories for two days a week.

Cons

1. You don't achieve a full fast

With this plan you do not completely abstain from food on your fasting days which also may result in you experiencing a rise in blood sugar during your fast. This may actually stall fat loss and reduce the pace at which you achieve your weight loss goals.

2. Adjusting to a full fast in future may be difficult

Some participants in this method of restricting calories to 500 per day on those days have reported that this actually makes them feel hungrier. This is said to make the adjustment to a period of complete fasting (as you progress) harder than if you adopted a method with a fasting period rather than a calorie restricting period to begin with.

3. Calorie counting

To make this plan effective, you will need to restrict your calories on your fasting days to around 500. This would involve being aware of how many calories each meal is which could prove to be a hassle to keep on top of.

Eat Stop Eat Method

There are various ways to implement intermittent fasting methods into your daily routine, but the Eat Stop Eat contains almost everything you need to stay healthy and manage your weight. This method is an effective way to shed off unnecessary weight and enhance the process of metabolism.

This method is similar to the 5:2 method with a slight adjustment. With the 5:2 method you restrict your calories for two of the five days in a week. With the Eat Stop Eat method, you are doing a full fast for two days within a week. All you need to do is choose one or two days of the week (never consecutive), during which you will completely abstain from eating for a complete 24 hours. It is important to know that for the remaining 5-6 days, you can eat whatever you want to eat. But you should make sensible food choices and avoid eating more than the necessary food that your body needs.

How to do this

The key to this type of plan is to stick to a full 24 hour fast. You can choose to fast for one day or two days weekly. When you choose to fast once a week, you can fast on Monday and eat for the rest of the week. If it's for two days, you can fast on Wednesday and Sunday, and eat the rest of the week. This method of fasting may be extremely challenging as an option. To make it slightly more achievable you could eat breakfast before 8 am on Monday and not eat until after 8 am on Tuesday for example. Once you feel comfortable with this method you could eliminate the breakfast before your fasting begins to make it more challenging and increase your fasting window. This is a completely optional addition to this method of IF.

Keep in mind that you need to drink more water when you are on the Eat Stop Eat method to keep your body hydrated, especially on your fasting days.

Days	Morning 8 am	Noon	Night
Monday	Eat (before 8 am)	Skip meal	Skip meal
Tuesday	Eat (after 8 am)	Eat	Eat
Wednesday	Eat	Eat	Eat
Thursday	Eat	Eat	Eat

Friday	Eat (before 8 am)	Skip meal	Skip meal
Saturday	Eat (after 8 am)	Eat	Eat
Sunday	Eat	Eat	Eat

Pros

Implementing the Eat Stop Eat method into your weekly routine gives you many advantages. You can be sure all those unnecessary fats are shed off, and a good body shape is maintained.

1. **Easy to follow**

This plan is not complicated and is really easy to follow.

2. **Backed by research**

Brad Pilon developed this method and there is mounting evidence that supports the claims that this method of fasting promotes weight loss more so than traditional forms of fasting.

3. **Inflammatory markers are lowered**

Chronic inflammation is linked to many debilitating diseases and the shift that the body has to endure with this method of fasting causes these inflammatory markers to be much lower.

Cons

Although this method is likely safe for women above fifty, it is essential to know some drawbacks. This method is not recommended for those beginning their IF journey, but may be one to consider as you become more adept to the concept of intermittent fasting. As mentioned before, always consult your doctor to give you peace of mind.

1. Insufficient nutrient intake

Fulfilling the nutritious requirement of this type of fasting may be really demanding. You may have to eat some high-protein and high-fiber foods that contain nutritious content to help you through this.

2. Self-Control

No matter how experienced you may be when it comes to fasting, being able to fast for 24 hours can be really tough to do consistently.

3. Adjustment period

Experts advise that participants of this form of fasting may experience side effects of mood swings, fatigue and dizziness at the adoption stage of this method. Your body needs to get used to using ketones instead of glucose as a source of energy.

How to Know Which One is Right for You

There are a few more variations of IF such as The Warrior Diet, Alternate Day Fasting and Meal Skipping. Although they all provide some merit and may be worth looking into, the methods we have just explored will provide you with the results you need as you begin IF. The methods we haven't explored are either too extreme or are only a slight variation of the methods we have already looked into. Even without them, you may be thinking, I have no idea where to start!

The key is to start slow, and it is acceptable if you decide to tweak the plan slightly to accommodate your lifestyle.

Another key you need to master when you are on any plan is consistency. You are likely to get the best result you want if you stick to a method for a long period. Sticking to intermittent fasting for a long time helps you to break away from certain eating habits.

Let's conclude with an extract from the Prime Women's website. "As with any diet, you'll get the best results if you're consistent. At the same time, you can certainly give yourself a break from this kind of eating schedule on special occasions. You should experiment to figure out which kind of intermittent fasting works the best for you. Lots of people ease themselves into IF with the 12-12 plan, and then they progress to 16-8. After that, you should try to stick to that plan as much as possible."

What Will Break My Fast?

This is extremely important to understand and grasp if you want to make the most of whatever schedule you decide to take on. There are various myths and unfounded theories on what you can and cannot eat/drink in your fasting period. The scientific research and studies around insulin and the reaction our bodies have to consuming certain snacks or food is growing and there are some seemingly creative ways to enhance taste without breaking your fast. Your blood sugar rises immediately after eating a meal or a snack and essentially puts the brakes on your body burning fat for fuel and turns on the signal to start storing incoming food mainly as fat (M. D. Jensen, M. Caruso, V. Hailing, and J. M. Miles). With this in mind, technically any intake of calories no matter how small either through sweeteners, a splash of milk in your coffee or a slice of fruit would break your fast because it would create a spike in your blood sugar levels and trigger food storage which is counterproductive to fast loss. An easy way to make sure you don't break your fast is always check what you are consuming has a zero calorie count, try to keep your fasting period simple with the beverages you choose to consume (water, black coffee, unsweetened tea with no milk). This will make sure you keep yourself in a fasted state without unknowingly instructing your body to store fat by spiking your insulin with 'fast breaking' type foods.

How You Should Break Your Fast

When you first start intermittent fasting you may be tempted to let the floodgates open when your feasting period begins. The thought of being able to eat after 12-16 hours feels like a reprieve worth taking advantage of with the largest meal you can muster up! The best way to break your fast however is to ease into it and not overwhelm your digestive system. Breaking your fast with snacks or foods high in sugar or fibre may result in bloating and discomfort (NLM).

The best way to break your fast is to ease into it with foods your digestive system can process easily without being shocked into overload. Below are a few fast breaking options worth considering when you decide to break your fast:

- **Smoothies** - A gentle way of introducing raw foods into the system.

- **Dried fruits** - A concentrated form of nutrients which will not overload your digestive system
- **Soups-** Another 'soft' introduction for your digestive system back to processing foods.

What Happens When Your Weight Loss Plateaus?

One of the frustrations you may experience regardless of the plan you choose is your weight loss beginning to plateau. Normally, your weight loss results in the first few months are really positive as your body reacts to the changes and deficit in calorie consumption. An article written in the Dietary Guidelines through researching weight loss plateau advises that typically this can happen around the *'6 month mark'* for most people. The body however is extremely intuitive and what may start to happen is the results you experienced at the beginning of your journey may begin to taper off. Theories around why this happen have been said to be down to the following;

- The body naturally adapts and defends itself against weight loss
- Participants stop following their plan as closely as they did to start with
- The metabolism slows down if you lose weight really quickly
- You are not creating a 'calorie deficit' by overeating
- Not enough exercise if any
- You have been on the same plan/routine for too long
- You are eating foods that contain counterproductive substances

The truth is that your weight loss can plateau even if you are following a plan consistently. This is common not only for women over 50, but for almost everyone attempting to lose weight over a prolonged period of time. Your body may start getting used to the plan you are on and begin to adapt and 'normalise' to the changes you have imposed. The key when this starts to happen is to make an adjustment. Assess the ratio of your IF method, change some of the recipes/food you intake or add in some exercise routines. You also have the option of modifying the intensity of those routines. Keep tweaking elements of your plan and measure your results (which we will detail later in the book) until you find an adjustment that kick starts the pursuit of your goals again. This will keep your metabolism on its toes and instruct your body to continue in the reduction of health repair and weight loss. One thing to consider is your metabolism. Naturally a high metabolism allows the body to burn calories at a much faster rate than someone whose metabolism is slightly slower. A person with low or slower metabolism will burn fewer calories at rest and during activity and therefore would have to eat less to counterbalance a sluggish metabolism. I know the frustration sometimes when I have come across people who tend to eat whatever they like and never seem to put the weight on!

As we develop in age, on average metabolism slows down which means that weight loss plateaus are almost inevitable and if you are following all the right steps laid out in this book and your weight loss stalls, do not be discouraged. Progress may seem like it's stalled externally but internally the recycling of old and damaged cells through the process of autophagy, the restraint and control you are developing and internal organ repairs taking place because of intermittent fasting are not immediately obvious, but it is continuously happening and never a waste to build upon. This is why getting your bloods done (later in this chapter) is a really helpful tool that will give you a snapshot of your internal health which is just as measurable and important as what the scale deems as progress.

Ditch The Scale!

The scale can be your best friend and your worst enemy, depending on what it tells you when you use it. The scale has always been a part of diets as the go to tool to determine if you have passed or failed. Similar to the days we have all experienced doing tests and waiting for our results to be communicated back. That sick feeling knowing you have cut corners and didn't expect good results or knowing you've worked hard and the results are returned and aren't what you expected. Sometimes the results are great and the motivation to continually work hard grows with every 'test' on the scale. Although our bodies are predictable to a degree with the heaps of studies and trials over the years underpinned by research and advocated by various nutritionists, life has a habit of getting in the way sometimes by hampering weight loss results. The curve balls we sometimes face show themselves through the makeup of your metabolism, health deficiencies, illness, family tragedies and so many other variables you just cannot account for. Whatever may get in the way or hinder your progress, the truth is if the scale doesn't reflect your desired results it can be extremely discouraging. This is why so many give up. A sense of guilt and dissolution sweeps through the mind and the point of you continuing doesn't seem worth it anymore. Sometimes, it's worth ditching the scale!

Now, this is not a headline to encourage you to ignore the fact you're not losing weight and not use the scale to bury your head in the sand. The scale is not always the most accurate method of measuring progress. Kate Heimburger, a physiologist based in Atlanta advises that 'a pound of fat weighs the same as a pound of muscle'. So if you are exercising and eating food that promotes muscle growth while intermittent fasting, you may be replacing the weight of some of your fat that's been reduced with the weight of muscle gain. The scale therefore would tell you haven't lost much weight when in reality you may have put on some muscle, which counterbalances the weight you would have lost if it was purely fat that had reduced! Even if this is not the case and your weight loss has drastically slowed down, as mentioned in the segment above getting your bloods done will give you a real feel of the progress you're making on the inside. Weight loss may be the catalyst for your journey but don't let it be an isolated motivating factor because of the endless variables that may affect the perceived progress of weight loss. Be sure to take into account how you feel, your mental progress, your energy levels and if the jeans you used to fit into can be worn now. Look in the mirror more often, be proud you have cut out late night snacking and give yourself credit for being healthier than you were before you started even if the scales don't always give you that credit. These are much healthier, sustainable long-term indicators of your overall progress!

Water Intake

Let's face it, water isn't the sexiest thing to talk about. Tasteless glasses of nothingness (seemingly) is a hard sell, especially when we have so many other variants of more appealing drinks to choose from. Thousands of different bottled flavoured water has been advertised which does taste better than more 'boring' bottles of natural water, but most of the time these 'water' variants are packed with sugar which actually minimises the benefits when you consume it and would also break your fast if you chose to have it in your fasting period. I may tell you something you may not want to hear; unflavoured natural water is *good for you and absolutely essential.* Nothing ground breaking, you may already know this, but it's worth reiterating because without water, the benefits of intermittent fasting are considerably diluted (pun very much intended). Water actually:

- Aids weight loss

- Keeps you hydrated
- Improves digestion
- Optimises kidney function

A study done in 2014 detailed in the Journal of Natural Science, Biology and Medicine on 50 overweight females, tasked them to drink 500 ml of water half an hour before breakfast, lunch, and dinner, in addition to their regular water consumption, for 8 consecutive weeks. All of those who participated experienced suppression in their appetite and a reduction in body weight, body fat, and BMI. A similar study detailed in the Journal of Clinical and Diagnostic Research demonstrated identical results. Besides the key benefits of hydration and digestion improvement, water suppressing the appetite is a fantastic way to maintain your fast in your restricted period.

How to Drink More Water

One of the most under-appreciated areas that need attention when you take on any IF plan, is your water intake. If this is not an area you generally struggle with, then continue with your good habit and drink as much water as you can. However, if you are like the majority of people and the required 8 glasses of water a day is not in your routine currently, then the following tips will help in developing this essential habit while you're fasting. One of the main enhancers of the side effects you may experience while intermittent fasting is dehydration and no surprise, water is the answer to reducing a lot of the side effects intensity.

Know your fluid needs

Just as there is a certain amount of calories that the body should take into avoiding malnutrition, there is a necessary amount of fluids that must get into your body over a period of time. One of the fluids that we have is water, and you can drink it to meet the needs of the body. You should make decisions about drinking more or less water based on your body's fluid needs. A popular recommendation is that all individuals should have a daily water intake of 2 litres or 8 cups.

Have a daily goal

You can increase your water intake if you set an active daily target. The word active here means that the goal you set for yourself should be acted upon. However, the act of setting a goal can act as motivation and increase your chances to make changes that would last for a long time. Ensure that the goals that you set gives you the best chance of success. If you want to be effective, ensure that the goals you set are smart; this means they must be specific, measurable, attainable, realistic, and time-bound. For example, you may be really enthusiastic and set a goal of 15 cups to drink daily; you might not be able to meet it unless you are living in the desert! A smart water-consumption goal can be to drink 2 litres daily (8 glasses), which is very achievable. If you have goals like this, it is easier to record your progress which increases your motivation and drives you to achieve that goal. The aim of a smart goal is to eventually become a subconscious habit.

Set reminders

The improvements in technology can also make it easy to take in more fluids. You can use your smartphone or a smartwatch to set reminders via an application or an alarm. For example, you can set a reminder that tells you to drink water every hour, and it could also be to remind you to finish your current water bottle and to refill after use. Such reminders can help you to increase the amount of water you drink daily, especially if you constantly forget to drink or you are too busy. There are a multitude of apps such as

Hydro Coach, Water Minder and many others that will automatically send you reminders to drink more water as opposed to you setting your own timer.

Replace other drinks with water

Another way that you can help you drink more water and improve your health without losing your objective of fasting intermittently, is to substitute other drinks which are not beneficial with water. Such drinks could be soda, sports drinks, and carbonated drinks because these drinks are often full of added sugars. The branding of these drinks can sometimes deceive us into thinking they do not contribute as much as they actually do to weight gain. Most commercialised drinks outside of water contain a surprisingly high amount of sugar. To put this into context, the table below illustrates how many teaspoons of sugar are in some of the most regularly consumed drinks amongst adults.

	Teaspoons	Calories
Soda (Fizzy Drinks)	11.5	185
Coca Cola	9.25	130
Sparkling Juice	5.5	110
Sports Drink	4	80
Bottled Ice Tea	7.5	109

Shocking, I know! Imagine putting nearly 10 teaspoons of sugar in your coffee? Well this is what you consume with every can of coke. If you can replace your regular intake of these drinks with water, you will be exposing your body to a completely new level of health and reduce the fats being created and stored by consuming all of that sugar. Incorporating this into your IF plan will help you shed that stubborn fat. It is difficult, no doubt about that. But so worth it for the results you will get by making this small change.

Drink water before each meal

I mentioned earlier that the aim of setting smart goals is for those actions to transform into habits. If you want to work towards achieving that goal with your actions, you can also create personal habits like drinking water before each meal. This would not only help you create a habit, but it will also help you to increase your water intake. If you eat four meals daily, it adds 4 cups to your daily water intake and you would be halfway to where you need to be. This also has an additional effect because many a time, your body might erroneously misjudge feelings of hunger with thirst, and drinking water would help to remove such dilemmas. When you drink water before you eat, you will be able to deduce what type of feeling it is. You should also know that drinking water during your intermittent fasting would also help to reduce the number of calories you will consume the next time you eat.

Flavour your water

Suppose you do not like how your water tastes, i.e., flavour; you can add a bit of flavour that can help you drink more water. There are a variety of flavour choices, such as fruit-infuser bottles, which are often inexpensive and healthy. You can use many fruit combinations in your fruit-infuser bottles, such as cucumber-lime, strawberry-kiwi, and lemon. You can use any kind of combination that suits your taste. There are also water enhancers that you can buy in liquid and powder form to add to your water, but most contain sugar. Bear in mind that flavouring your water this way while you are fasting *would break your fast* if you did it this way in your restricted period. However, you can use this method to help consume water during your feasting period and switch to normal unflavoured water while fasting.

Drink one cup of water every hour at work

You can make it a habit to drink water every hour that you spend at work. For example, if you have a 9 to 5 job where you work for 8 hours and drink water every hour, it adds 8 cups to your daily water intake. You can do this in the morning when you get to work and refill; repeat this process every hour throughout a workday, and you will have a consistent water intake.

Consume more foods that have high water content

Another way that you can use to meet your daily target is by eating more foods that are high in water content. Good sources of food with high water content are fruits and vegetables such as lettuce, honeydew melon, cabbage, celery, cantaloupe, and zucchini. In addition to high amounts of water in these fruits and vegetables, they are also packed with vitamins, antioxidants, and minerals that will improve your overall health.

What are Electrolytes?

Electrolytes is a popular buzzword for many in the weight loss space. Electrolytes are compounds that dissociate to form ions when they are dissolved in water. However, electrolytes in relation to the human body are more complicated than that. Here, electrolytes are the essential minerals present in the body's fluids. Examples of such fluids are blood, urine, and water. When the electrolytes minerals are dissolved, they create electrically charged ions. The ions that were created by these minerals act as catalysts for all of the functions in the body.

The electrically charged ions create pulses of electricity that can be likened to spark plugs for the cell. These ions also help to activate nerve and muscle functions. You should know that electrolytes make it possible for the vitamins obtained from food to exert their physiological influences. There are other important duties that electrolytes do in the human body.

Will electrolytes break your fast?

This is extremely key to understanding and making a clear distinction between which electrolytes break your fast and which do not is really simple. Minerals essentially have no energy value and pure electrolytes contain no calorie content or macronutrients. So do they break your fast? The answer is if you consume pure electrolytes then they do not. Most fasting salts or pure electrolyte products are readily available to purchase and these will not break your fast. There is electrolyte supplements specifically calibrated for fasting (fasting salts), which come in powder form (to be mixed with water) or in tablet form. Although they are advertised as pure, still check the labels and descriptions to make sure. There are however some products or supplements that may contain electrolytes but are not pure minerals and normally loaded with sweeteners, artificial flavours and fillers like maltodextrin. Obvious examples of this are sports drinks, which as you'd expect are filled with sugars and compiled with calories. It's important to check the labels, anything other than pure electrolytes (which contain zero calories and no added ingredients or additives) would break your fast, other than this, using unblemished electrolyte supplements is a fantastic way to aid you in your fasting schedule and maintain a healthy balance of minerals within your body without breaking your fast.

Do you need to increase your electrolyte consumption during fasting?

Generally, fasts that are considered 'shorter' are usually less than 48 hrs of continuous fasting. Any length of time beyond this timeframe would absolutely require some form of electrolyte support. Shorter fasts like OMAD or any variation of the 16:8 IF eating patterns would benefit from electrolyte support but it's not essential due to you having an opportunity to replenish electrolytes within a 24-hour period with food and water. Each individual is different and the makeup of our genetics play a role in what volume of electrolytes is naturally stored within our body.

How do I know I need more electrolytes?

There are a couple of ways to monitor your deficiencies and assess whether you may need to focus some attention on this aspect of your eating schedule. One way is getting your bloods checked which can be done by your local health practitioner or there are a variety of home testing kits that can be used. Like anything, the quality and accuracy of the home testing kits may vary and it may be worth making sure whoever you use is qualified and highly recommended through accreditations. Getting your blood screened is a great way to understand any deficiencies you may have (more on getting your bloods done later) and the areas you need to focus on. This is always a good starting point but it may not be a sustainable way of monitoring your mineral composition by regularly getting blood tests. Here is a breakdown of what may indicate you are in need of a balance of electrolytes:

Not enough electrolytes:

- Muscle cramps or weakness
- Headaches
- Fatigue

- Dizziness

- Nausea

- Brain fog

- Depression

- Irregular or fast heartbeat

Over consumption of electrolytes:

- Bloating

- Swollen ankles or fingers

- Stomach pain

- Diarrhoea

How many electrolytes should you consume?

We tend to get a fix of electrolytes through our daily water and food consumption and this component of our daily intake is usually misunderstood and relatively unknown. They form such a vital part of our body's function and fluidity that any sort of attention and focus placed on improving this aspect of your eating pattern will pay huge dividends in the long run. During a long fast, you are no longer consuming the electrolytes the body needs to function at its peak. Your body has a small reserve of electrolytes stored in its tissues but this usually depletes within the first 24-48 hrs of fasting. As soon as your body starts to detect a deficiency of electrolytes the body reacts with headaches, fatigue, muscle cramps, nausea and just generally not feeling great. This is because electrolytes are key in regulating your pH levels and muscles, keeping you hydrated and consuming a healthy dose and variation of electrolytes in your diet is extremely important for your health. This is why water is so important while fasting as it helps supplement some of the reduction of electrolytes through your calorie restriction and contributes to maintaining the balance our bodies are continuously aspiring to achieve. We naturally lose electrolytes when we sweat (Sodium), vomit or have diarrhea and lose key minerals that need to be replenished hence the common feelings of headaches, fatigue and that 'ughhh' worn out feeling you would have after these experiences. This is why replenishing electrolytes is recommended after workouts as we lose key minerals when we sweat and being able to replenish the loss of electrolytes through supplements is a great way to maintain a balance.

Can I over consume electrolytes?

For all the health benefits of electrolytes, it is important to note that like most things there is a balance to maintain. Over consuming some of these minerals can actually do more harm than good to your health. Many people unknowingly are over consuming some minerals through their current eating patterns, which can lead to some health complications. On most food and drink nutrition labels there are details of what value of electrolytes you will intake by consuming that food or beverage. The 'Daily Value' % or NRV's on the nutrition labels give you some guidance on the percentage of the Daily Value for each nutrient in a serving of the food or drink. Use this as a reference to understand how to combat some of the deficiencies you have and steer clear of over consuming some of these minerals especially Sodium which may contribute to high blood pressure if over consumed. Some of the common electrolytes found in the body and what the National Institute of Health (NIH) recommended daily limits are as follows:

- **Calcium** - 1,200 mg for females aged 51 years and older
- **Chloride** - Roughly 2,300 mg - Most consumption of Chloride is through salt.
- **Magnesium** - 320 mg for females 30 years +

- **Phosphorus -** 700 mg
- **Potassium -** 2,600 mg for adult females
- **Sodium -** Max of 2,300 mg

Some of these minerals are more common than others in your diet and you may have heard of electrolytes through the advertisement of sports drinks which is very common. Whilst there is truth in these drinks providing you with some of these minerals, these drinks are combined with high levels of sugar and dyes which clearly would be counterproductive. There are much more sustainable food and drinks that you can consume some of these key minerals through, here are just a few:

Spinach - An amazing source of magnesium 73% DV and calcium 23% DV combined with Vitamin A and Vitamin K.

Pickle Juice - Packed with sodium and chloride and commonly associated with the reduction is muscle spasms. Be careful not to over consume foods with sodium as too much of this mineral may lead to an increase in high blood pressure.

Lentils - Legumes have a huge amount of electrolytes and especially magnesium. They are really easy to incorporate into your diet with a variety of meals you can combine them in.

Dried Apricots - Not only are these sweet, tasty and a fantastic snack, half a cup of dried apricots have almost a quarter of the daily required value of potassium for adults.

Sunflower Seeds - These crunchy seeds are a great source of phosphorus and also share a similar value in magnesium as nuts.

Coconut Water – 240 g of unsweetened coconut water has a varied composition of electrolytes:

- 396 mg of potassium

- 16.8 mg of calcium

- 62.4 mg of sodium

- 14.4 mg of magnesium

Plant based Milk- Unsweetened Soya, Almond and Oat milk are fantastic sources of electrolytes and healthy dairy alternatives. Each of these have their own make up of electrolytes (Calcium, Sodium & Potassium) combined with minimal to no sugar, cholesterol and saturated fat. Cow's milk does offer comparable electrolyte components and research by the International Dairy Journey states *'not only do plant-based milks fail to provide comparable levels of vitamins and minerals, but the vitamins and minerals are absorbed less easily than those present in cow's milk too.* Whilst this may be true, cow's milk does contain much higher levels of cholesterol (24 mg), sugars (12 mg), carbohydrates (11 mg) and saturated fat (7 mg) per 250 ml cup according to the USDA. Conclusively, plant based dairy alternatives offer a much healthier, sustainable and varied composition of milk with vitamins and electrolytes than that of cow's milk.

Understand All the Categories of Sugar Alternatives

There are four popular types of sugar substitutes which are artificial sweeteners, novel sweeteners, natural sweeteners, and sugar alcohols. All categories have their benefits and disadvantages depending on the objective. Remember, sugar alternative will still break your fast if consumed during your feasting window as they carry calorie content.

Why is it important to reduce sugar?

There are many reasons why you should reduce your sugar intake. It could be because you are trying to reduce your calorie intake or as a result of health challenges. If you have diabetes, you should only take artificial sweeteners or sugar alcohols in moderate amounts as it is a better option.

Are sugar alternatives really a healthier option?

The effect of a sugar substitute in your body depends on which type of sweetener you use, the quantity you have used, and the reason why you use it.

Artificial sweeteners

These are synthetic sugar substitutes that have strong sweetening abilities, and you should only use them in small amounts to increase the flavour in food. The studies on artificial sweeteners and the effects on insulin levels have provided mixed results. Studies done by The National Library of Medicine have reported that 'artificial sweeteners are safe for diabetics' and will not raise your blood sugar levels. These studies have yet to be carried out on a long term trial and therefore the long term effects of artificial sweeteners on humans are relatively unknown. With that in mind, the following detail around sugar alternatives provides findings and details relating to sweeteners with all the relevant data we have to work with currently. Many of the sweeteners available have small studies that suggest that your blood sugar levels do not get raised through artificial sweeteners. This may be the case, but with the little research around this topic be sure to take this option up in moderation and with the awareness that future studies may shed more light on this area that would indicate more concrete results either for or against sugar substitutes. One thing that is clear, is that the health benefits of sweeteners far outweigh the benefits of sugar.

Novel sweeteners

It is difficult to characterize these sweeteners because they are derived from highly refined natural sources. An example is Stevia that has been researched and shown to have some health benefits like managing diabetes and reducing blood pressure.

Sugar alternatives

There are many substitutes of sugar that you can use, and here is a list to guide you on suitable sugar substitutes and how you can incorporate them into your diet.

Acesulfame potassium (Ace-K)

Ace-K is an artificial sweetener that does not cause tooth decay, increase blood sugar or increase calorie intake. You can use this by adding it to food at the table and it is also heat-stable. Its resistance to heat makes it a suitable option that can be used in cooking and baking. You can use it in beverages and it is 200 times sweeter than sugar. However, Ace-K does not provide the same bulk and volume as table sugar and ensures that you make an adjustment to your recipe when you use it.

Agave nectar

Agave nectar is a natural sweetener that supplies more nutrients than table sugar and less than honey. This sugar substitute is rich in flavour and you do not use it in large quantities. Agave nectar contains high amounts of calories and lots of fructose which can cause weight gain and obesity when you use it in high amounts. It is also sweeter than sugar and has a long shelf life. It is also heat-stable and can be substituted for other substitutes while cooking. It has a similar taste to honey but without the bitter aftertaste like some sugar substitutes. Whenever you use this sugar substitute, you might have to make modifications to your recipes because it is in liquid form.

Coconut sugar

Coconut sugar is also a natural sweetener that is unrefined. The unrefined nature means that it retains all vitamins and minerals and does not cause fluctuations in blood sugar. This sweetener contains the same amount of calories as table sugar. It is not a good option for diabetic patients, and you should limit it if you want to lose weight. You can use it as a direct replacement for white or brown sugar. It is very coarse, and you will have to grind it in a blender before you can use it in the kitchen.

Honey

Honey is a natural sweetener that has more nutrients than table sugar, including antioxidants, minerals, and vitamins. Honey is easily digestible in comparison with table sugar. Similar to table sugar, it is very high in calories and can be broken down into glucose and fructose, and poses some health challenges. You can use it in smoothies, sauces, baked goods, and sauces. You can also use it for cooking, but you should be careful about the amount you add since it is sweeter than sugar.

Monk fruit extracts

Monk fruit extracts are a healthy sugar substitute that you can use if you are trying to reduce calorie intake. It is a Novel sweetener, and you do not need to use it in large quantities since it is sweeter than sugar. According to the FDA, it does not add calories and has no side effects. However, some commercial products of these fruit extracts have sugar and sweeteners in them, which were added during their processing. You can use it in cooking and baking. This novel sweetener has an aftertaste and makes modifications to your cooking because it is very sweet.

Date paste

Date paste is a natural sweetener that is rich in minerals, fiber, and vitamins, which makes it more nutritious than regular sugar. It is easy to make; its ingredients are ¾ cup of water, 1 cup of warm pitted dates, and half a teaspoon of vanilla extract. You can use it in smoothies, marinades, salad dressings, sauces, and baked goods. It is sweeter than sugar; make modifications to your recipe to accommodate it.

Maple syrup

This syrup is rich in antioxidants rich in minerals like calcium, potassium, iron, manganese, and zinc. Maple syrup has high amounts of calories and should be consumed moderately. You can use it in many dishes besides its common use in pancakes and waffles. You can use it in healthier breakfast options like oatmeal and plain yogurt and in savory dishes like vegetables and salad dressings.

Stevia extracts

Stevia extracts are an HGH intensity novel sweetener derived from plant extracts that have little to no calories. You can use it if you are trying to control your weight, and it is also sweeter than sugar. There are many forms after it has been refined, and it has an aftertaste which makes it unsuitable for coffee and tea.

Sucralose

Sucralose, whose brand name is Splenda, is an artificial sweetener that does not have any calories. It is about 600 times sweeter than sugar, and it can be used by diabetic patients, pregnant women and breastfeeding mothers. If you are trying to restrict sugar, it is a good option. You should use sucralose in small amounts, especially when baking.

Xylitol

Xylitol is a sugar alcohol that contains low amounts of calories and is sweeter than sugar. These sugar substitutes do not promote tooth decay or cause a sudden increase in blood sugar. It is a very good option for people with diabetes, but it could have laxative effects like diarrhea and bloating when taken in large amounts. You can find it in chewing gum, jam, baked goods, and frozen yogurt. It can be used in place of sugar in fruit, cereal, and beverages.

The aim of intermittent fasting is to stay healthy and controlling your sugar intake can play a huge part in getting to the goals you set out. Refined sugar intake is the cause of many cases of weight gain and health related issues. If you have a sweet tooth and need your sugar fix, try some of these replacements and you're likely to still enjoy the sweetness you crave without the damage that comes with refined sugar.

Blood Screening

Getting your bloods proactively checked is not something that most people would do outside of it being requested by your doctor or health practitioner. The reason this tends to be requested is because getting your blood checked can provide extremely accurate indications of what is going on inside of our bodies and give context to why we feel the way we do sometimes. Getting your blood screened will give you a screenshot of your current state of health and potentially catch health problems before they rise to the surface. In general, blood tests can reveal:

- The current state of your internal health
- See how well your internal organs are working (e.g. kidney, liver)
- Gauge risk of heart disease
- Detail any mineral deficiencies
- Assess how your body deals with inflammation, infection and injury
- Checks cholesterol and glucose levels

How is this relevant to intermittent fasting? Beyond the immediate and obvious benefits of your wider health being assessed, having your bloods checked can give you important data to work with while intermittent fasting. Your weight may be an external catalyst to take intermittent fasting on, however there may be deficiencies, degenerative diseases and root causes to health issues that the blood test could pick up and this could give you areas of your health you could use intermittent fasting to focus on and improve. While this is not essential for you to do when starting intermittent fasting, understanding any mineral deficiencies, internal organ problems, inflammation markers etc. is useful knowledge to have and incorporate measures into your intermittent fasting schedule (electrolytes, specific foods etc.) to help reduce any health risks. In addition, sometimes you may not lose as much weight through IF as you would have liked despite following the plan and eating healthy as you potentially hit a plateau in weight loss. What you may find is that a lot of the benefits accrued through IF is actually done internally through lowering your cholesterol, infection and diabetes risk, which will not show up on the scale, but this progress will be demonstrated through your blood test results.

Where You can Get Blood Screening Done

The most common place to get this done would be through your doctor, but there are now many more accessible home testing kids that have the results tested and provided by accredited health practitioners. Here are a couple worth having a look at:

Thriva (only available in the UK)

This company has an app you can download and input what you want checked within your blood. A home testing kit is sent to you with a huge amount of detail and really easy instructions to follow. The results are relayed back to you within a couple of days with descriptive context detailed within the app against each element tested for. Thriva also provides a plan and suggestions on how to improve specific aspects of your health where your blood indicates there may be deficiencies.

Let's Get Checked (Available in the USA and various countries)

A health diagnostics company started in 2014 that gives the options to check a multitude of health related concerns through home testing kits. Heart health, cancer screening, digestive health and mineral deficiencies are just a few of the areas that can be tested. If any of the tests come back with concerning results, a free consultation is offered with a nurse to discuss the best way forward to tackle any issues. Usually all of your results are produced within a couple of days.

To some this option may seem excessive; it's certainly not mandatory. It is however a practice that can provide you insight into your health that wasn't as accessible a few years ago as it is today. With affordable home testing kits, you can get some real data that could not only help you avoid health related pitfalls, you will have fantastic data to use as a reference point in your health journey. I completely get that this topic is a side step from IF, its benefits and how to implement an eating schedule. However, there is no harm in exploring various tools that could help aid your understanding of your health as a whole and use that within your IF implementation.

Checklist

- Choose a schedule that works for you and a ratio to start with
- Understand why your weight loss may plateau and what tweaks you can make if that happens
- Set water intake reminders or download a suitable app to assist you
- Reduce sugar intake and use a suggested replacement
- Look into blood screening/work options.

Chapter Three:

Losing Weight the Right Way

It's one thing to understand a routine, it's another to actually stick to it. How often do you see these amazing weight loss stories and pictures of women who have lost so much weight and look amazing? Transformational before and after photos seem like they could never contain pictures of you. You have tried before and nothing seems to work, so why is this different? The reason IF is so well received is because of the results women have had when they have fully committed to it. However, for the majority of us, it is difficult to stick to a routine that feels like such a step change from our normal daily lives. Food is a constant in every person's life and IF, or any weight loss regime may seem like an imposter.

This is why the next few chapters are so important. The information we will go through will give you all the best possible tools to help you get the most out of intermittent fasting and lose weight the right way. Setting realistic goals, how to measure weight vs muscle loss; which is all critical detail that will not only aid your weight loss but sustain it through long term habits with measurable results. Later on, we will also delve into exercise tips, useful apps, videos and conclude with some amazing recipes specifically constructed to achieve certain results. Before we get there, let's stick to the topic at hand.

The pancreas produces a hormone called insulin in your body. This hormone helps convert glucose (sugar) in your body to the energy that your cells need for proper functioning. Insulin also aids fat storage. This insulin level increases during non-fasting days but decreases during fasting days. In other words, the insulin level is lower during the fasting period but increases during eating time. More insufficient insulin during fasting can help prevent additional fat storage and help the body use and burn the stored fat.

When you engage with a method of IF and stick to the plan, you should expect a good weight loss of about 3-5 kg's per month. This is an estimate based on a multitude of biological variables and the composition of your body specifically. What you will need to be mindful of is how much of the weight you are losing is fat vs muscle. Muscle loss can be dangerous, but absolutely avoidable with the right attentiveness and monitoring.

Muscle Loss vs. Fat Loss

At this point, it is essential to know that there is a dime's worth of differences between muscle loss and fat loss. Many people think they are the same and it can be hard to differentiate when you are losing fat and when you are losing muscle. Knowing the difference between the two will give you the confidence that the loss in weight is fat and not muscle that you need to retain.

Losing muscle can be damaging, as it is one of the vital components of your overall health. When you maintain healthy muscle, you have several benefits;

- Maintain healthy fat levels

70

- Retain healthy sugar levels
- Control inflammation
- Strength and stability

More so, you may likely reduce the risk of age-related muscle loss that can lead to permanent disabilities or weakness if you maintain a healthy muscle mass. One really cool benefit of having a healthy amount of muscle mass is the more muscle you have, the more calories you burn when you nap. Muscle tissue is metabolically more active and burns more calories than fat tissue (Rolfe & Brown, 1997). The higher your muscle mass, the bigger your resting energy expenditure and in turn your body will burn more calories while you are not active (sleeping, resting etc.). This is not an endorsement to become a bodybuilder, but there are passive benefits of maintaining muscle mass. This reinforces why careful attention should be paid on how to lose fat but maintain or gain more muscle.

Those who want to lose weight sometimes do not consider muscle growth, but the role that muscle mass plays in weight loss is significant. Before you consider picking up the largest weights you can find and aspire to bench press like Arnold Schwarzenegger, referring back to earlier in the book a study found that most women will experience muscle loss of up to 40% by the time they get to 80 years old. This loss in muscle mass also plays a part in the rate that weight loss occurs due to lack thereof. So while we may look at ways to measure and avoid unnecessary muscle mass loss, always try to incorporate high protein based foods and exercise routines into your plan to promote muscle gain and the by-product of this will be accelerated weight loss.

To maintain or gain muscle, constantly practice exercising, eat plenty of high protein foods, and follow a plan that reduces your calorie intake. The bottom line is this: while weight loss is all about reducing your overall weight, fat loss refers to weight loss resulting from failures in fat mass. That's why you should prioritize losing weight in the form of fat instead of muscle. Don't panic! There are ways you can measure and monitor to make sure that the loss of weight you will experience is the right type of weight loss.

How to Take Measurement

Taking a measurement is perhaps the most reliable, effective, and flexible way of tracking your progress when adopting a weight loss strategy. Unfortunately, relying on a scale for measurement is not the most accurate way of determining the quality of your results. The scale takes into consideration every glass of water, snack and morsel of food consumed. There is no way of differentiating what you are gaining, which could just be water, or losing which also could be water.

How to Measure Yourself during Intermittent Fasting

Few things are important to keep in mind when you measure yourself during fasting. However, it would help if you took note of the following to get the desired result you want.

- Stand with your feet together
- Relax your body for the measurement
- Have an inelastic or flexible tape (a cloth measuring tape is preferable)
- For accuracy, ensure you do your measurement twice, immediately after the first time.
- Then, take the average of both measurements to get the final result.

Where to Measure

Every person's body composition is completely different and there is no way to distribute fat to one area and not the other. The key to these measurements is to keep track of your body composition and make sure that the muscle you have is not being compromised. Here is where part of the body you should measure:

Abs: To measure your abs, stand and ensure your feet are tightly together and your torso straight but relaxed.

Hips: To accurately measure your hips, you need to get a mirror. Try looking in the mirror while standing sideways. Ensure the tape is parallel to the ground.

Waist: Measure your natural waist or the narrowest part of your torso.

Arms: Stand straight and ensure one arm is relaxed. Then, find the midpoint between the shoulder bone and the elbow of that arm.

Thighs: Measure the midpoint between the lower part of your glutes and the back of your knees.

Calves: Measure halfway between knees and the ankle.

It's advisable to measure yourself every week for the first month or so of your journey and bi-weekly thereafter. The best time to do these measurements is first thing in the morning before you eat or drink anything. Try and keep the routine of your measurements the same to have reliable results.

How to do Body Fat Measurement

As a woman above fifty, there are different ways you can measure your body fat. But you should realize that some are more reliable and accurate than others. There are 'body fat scales' that use a technology called bioelectrical impedance analysis (BIA). These scales vary in price, however, accuracy can be questionable with these pieces of hardware. Calipers are also a traditional way to measure body fat and provide the most cost effective and fastest results.

Setting Realistic Goals for Losing Weight

Weight loss goals vary from person to person. Your weight loss goal is different from your friend's, and hers is different from yours. It is important that you choose a goal that is medically safe and effective, which you can incorporate into a long-term dieting plan.

According to the Centers for Disease Control and Prevention, women above fifty are advised that in order to lose weight effectively through IF you must set *'weekly, achievable and realistic goals'*. The goals for losing weight are one to two pounds per week. The Center further reported that women who lost weight at that pace might likely continue to lose weight for a long time. To reach the goal, you should reduce your calorie intake by 500 to 1,000 daily. This is because one pound of body fat is summed to be 3,500 calories.

If you have obesity-related conditions at your age, following a low-calorie diet will be helpful. In addition, it would help you to reduce the risk of health conditions such as high blood pressure, cholesterol, heart diseases, and diabetes.

According to Weight-loss Information Network, obese women can lose 3 to 5 pounds weekly if they adopt low-calorie diets that contain 800 or fewer calories per day. However, it is good you know that adopting very-low-calorie diets comes with risk. Nevertheless, they are helpful and recommendable when you are under the supervision of an expert or a healthcare provider.

You Can Meet Your Goals with Weight Loss Apps

There is no blanket approach to how you chose to incorporate IF. The plans within the IF portfolio are a framework and the aids you use within the schedule to help you get to your goals is completely down to you. Most apps today are based on traditional dieting or have an underlying weight loss approach. That being said, apps can be really useful in helping monitor your calorie intake, provide tailored recipes or just be a means of keeping track of your progress.

Having an app to track your progress is certainly not essential. Following an IF plan and eating healthy will get amazing results on their own. However, the use of user-friendly apps for self-monitoring is an excellent and effective way to increase the awareness of your habits and track your progress.

Here are a selection of apps that could be useful to consider but are by no means essential. Most of these apps are free but the nature of this space is that things are likely to change. Have a look at the detail below and see if any would be useful to achieving your goals.

Window- Intermittent fasting

Window is a highly recommended app specifically targeted for beginners starting their IF journey. You can easily set up your scheduled eating windows, allow notifications to remind you when your eating window is open or closed and you can also sync it to the Apple Health app.

There are also some really handy in App recommendations on how to be a healthier version of yourself, gets a thumbs up from me! There is a paid for premium version of the app where you can add more detail and be a bit more hands on by attaching daily notes, photos and track your weight. *'If you're unsure where to begin, the Windows app can really help with that, it can keep you motivated with the visuals'* Colleen Moltzen, a registered dietitian at Keatley MTN.

Fastic

We have touched on fasting being more than just 'not eating'. It is so much more than that! Fastic not only has some really cool features that help you monitor your progress and windows opening and closing, there are over 400 amazing recipes to choose from. The recipes are all healthy, filling and intentionally designed for those who are fasting and need good wholesome food to enhance your chances of reaching your goals.

One of the really helpful features is the fasting community you will get access to via the app. You'll be able to engage and communicate with a large group of fasters within the app to help you in your journey.

Zero

If you have customised your eating schedule and it falls outside of the standard structure we have gone through in this book. It may be difficult to keep track of when you are supposed to eat and when you are not. Zero allows you customise the tracking of your eating windows so you get reminders at exactly when the right time to either start or break your fast will be. You can also choose from several preset fasting windows or create your own personalised one lasting up to seven days. A nice simple and clean design with a dashboard that is not filled with confusing information, a nice app to start with!

Fastient

Tracking your fasting times and monitoring your diet could not be easier with Fastient. This app is definitely one of the more comprehensive tracking apps available with features that allow you to maintain a record of your food intake and keep tabs on your overall progress all in one place. A large, clean interface with plenty of space to record and review your personal data in graphs and charts with access available on your phone or desktop. *"When it comes to following a meal plan for results, tracking is key for progress and accountability," Erin Palinski-Wade – RD, CDE*

BodyFast

This application attempts to take a scientific based approach to the IF schedules. You will get a lot of the features described in the apps above, however BodyFast will also give you 10 different fasting plans to choose from. There are also loads of helpful tips and advice as well as coaching notes that can be found.

One thing to consider with this app, the coaching is automated based on the data you input around age, weight etc. It doesn't take into consideration variants like medication, body composition and other factors that may skew the advice being relevant to your unique situation. Always take into consideration the advice you have been given by either a dietician or medical practitioner who knows your medical history and body composition better than anyone.

There are some other really good apps out there such as Vora, FastHabit and LIFE Fasting tracker, however everything you need to get started will be found in any one of the apps we just went through. The apps will be really useful to you if you know what you want to achieve and you are specific about it. The next section will talk you through how to set up SMART goals and these apps can be an aid in helping you achieve every aspect of your goals.

How Can SMART Goals be Helpful?

As a woman above fifty, it's incredibly important to set goals when you want to try any method of intermittent fasting. Goals help provide clarity of purpose, and they give you focus. But there is a smart way to write goals and objectives on intermittent fasting that you probably need to know.

There is something powerful about setting a goal and achieving it. One of the biggest mistakes we have all made is spur of the moment goals that are fuelled by such a strong desire to change that the bar of achievement gets set too high. Intentions can be good and lofty goals have their place, but in order to stay motivated they need to be considered and achievable. Remember, the body you want to have or the person you want to become doesn't have to be achieved in one attempt. You can get there with multiple, small, achievable goals along the way. Every goal achieved will give you confidence and motivation to carry on and achieve even more until eventually, you are exactly where you want to be. The perception of failing to achieve the results we set out to achieve is the biggest destroyer of progression. This is where SMART goals can help.

SMART is the acronyms for specific, measurable, achievable, realistic, and timely. These are components that your goal should have. Women who have set un-SMART goals can tell you how frustrating and draining and unrealistic the pursuit for weight loss and overall health through intermittent fasting can be. Most of us are quick to decide what we want, but we never take time to organize our ideas and arrange them so that they would be specific, measurable, and achievable within a time frame.

Using the SMART goals method for intermittent fasting makes it easy for you to achieve your daily or weekly goals. For example, if your goal is to lose weight, you should set a goal like: "By the end of next month, I should have lost 5 pounds." Once you have done this you can break your monthly goal into a weekly one, 1.25 pounds per week. This will give you a clearly defined measurable goal you can monitor weekly and track your progress. Remember to start with a realistic goal, one that gives you every chance to achieve and breed confidence for the next goal you set.

Now, let's study how the SMART goal formula will help you clarify and create new and improved goals. Replicate each SMART category onto your own piece of paper and tailor each section to your personal goals for the results you want.

GOAL: I want to lose weight.

Specific: I _will_ lose (choose a specific amount of weight you want to lose). Be as specific as you can and this will give you a clear and defined target to hit.

Measurable: Use a scale or measuring tape to keep track of your weight loss journey and note it down every week. Have a set day and time in the week to take measurements and be as consistent as you can to give yourself the most accurate information to measure your progression.

Achievable: Use a dress or a piece of clothing you used to be able to fit into as a target of where you want to be. Make sure your goals are achievable. Take into consideration your lifestyle, work patterns etc. to attain the weight loss results and make sure it's an achievable goal.

Relevant: Why is it important to you to lose weight? Everyone has different motivations for doing so. Some women just want to be healthier, feel better about the way they look or just get rid of stubborn belly fat. Whatever your motivation, be clear of what it is from the start and refer back to it when you inevitably have a wobble in your weight loss journey.

Time-Bound: Set a timeframe to keep yourself honest and have an end point you can work towards. A good starting point is 30 days.

When you are done setting the goals, go through them and write them according to each SMART feature, you can then put together all the work you have done into one SMART goal. With that, you can be sure that your goals will be achieved within the time frame you have set for them.

In sum, you have learned how you can lose weight the right way. You know what you need to lose between muscle and fat. Absolutely, your understanding of why and how to measure your progress when you are intermittent fasting has been enhanced. Also, you are now familiar with some mobile apps that can help you track your calorie intake and monitor you until your dietary goal is achieved. Ultimately, you can now set goals – SMART goals and follow through until you reach your goal.

Checklist

- Make sure you measure yourself to avoid muscle loss
- Chose an App to aid and motivate you through the process

- Write down and tailor the SMART goals to reflect what outcome you desire
- Are your goals realistic?

Chapter Four:

Exercise That You Can Do At Home

The dreaded eight letter word- exercise. I am almost certain that every person reading this book has flirted with exercise to some degree. I have been through countless phases of getting into a routine of exercising and keeping active, only for it to taper off and eventually never happen again. I would convince myself that I'd eventually get back to it, maybe tomorrow, actually, wouldn't it be better to start on a Monday? Yes, it makes absolute sense to delay having to face putting my body through stress for another week but I was sure I would be ready come Monday. The day would come and I would find another excuse- no shock there!

Intermittent fasting alone may be enough for some to slim down, control eating habits or achieve whatever health related goal without a dedicated exercise routine being part of the schedule. Remember, your body is naturally burning calories through your normal daily activities such as cleaning your house, walking your dog and even through sex. With a change in your diet and an increase in some of the daily activities mentioned (I'll leave it to you to decide which ones) you may find that being a good place to start. The key thing is to start with steps that feel like a natural progression because a sudden commitment to exercise 3 days a week with intermittent fasting being brand new to you, will increase the chances of you burning out. This advice might sound counterproductive to most books that would encourage you to dive into IF, limit your eating to small windows for seven days, add three days in of one hour exercise sessions and only eat new recipes you've never attempted before- sounds a bit overwhelming right? 10% of something is better than 100% of nothing. Small carefully planned steps of progression are better than not doing anything at all because not everyone is comfortable with making wholesale changes right from the beginning.

There is no doubt however, that dedicated exercise for women over 50 has huge benefits and introducing exercise into your plans eventually is highly advisable. Once you get to grips with IF as a routine, within the first 30 days would be a really good place to start implementing a workout routine. Like many other women who have followed the guidelines of IF, you will notice weight loss, but as we discussed earlier in the book there is a fine line between weight loss and muscle loss. The measuring methods discussed in the previous chapter will help you monitor that decrease but exercise will help counter muscle loss by targeting muscle growth. *'You lose muscle as you get older, exercise helps you rebuild it'* (*The National Institute of Ageing*)

Exercising is the traditionally accepted means when discussing weight loss. However, your diet and eating patterns are arguably even more important than any exercise routine. This may be true, but a balance is needed. Being over 50, the importance of not losing muscle is critical and any attempt to lose weight may also spill over into muscle loss if some exercise to strengthen your muscles is not implemented into your routine. Don't start running to the gym to renew your membership just yet, there are some simple and effective exercises you can do in the comfort of your own home.

Generally there are three categories when it comes to exercising;

- **Cardio** - This involves increasing your heart rate which builds endurance and burns calories. E.g. Running, swimming and walking.
- **Strength or Weight Training** - Increases muscle growth and strength, e.g. exercising with weights or resistance training.
- **Flexibility** - Promotes a limber body that is more resistant to injury e.g. stretching and yoga.

First, let's start with how exercising can help accelerate your desired results.

How Exercise Can Accelerate Your Slimming Process While Fasting

With intermittent fasting, you aim to be healthy and strong while you rock your fifties in style. When you combine exercise with your intermittent fasting plan, you can get accelerated slimming results while you maintain a healthy status. You don't have to worry about losing muscles, and you can gain and maintain a healthy muscle mass for many years to come with a steady resistance based exercise routine.

How Much Do You Need to Exercise Weekly?

This will depend on varying factors as everyone does not age the same and physical limitations differ. According to studies done across participants over fifty, 150 minutes of moderate exercise five days a week or 75 minutes of vigorous exercise is considered a good amount of activity. This doesn't take into consideration any fasting or calorie restriction being applied by the participant. When you first start IF, your body will be experiencing a bit of a shock to the system. You are now taking control and telling your body when to expect food as opposed to your body dictating when you should eat. Naturally, your body will resist this change in defense of it's routine through the side effects we discussed earlier in the book. You may not have as much energy as you normally would and feel a bit weaker as you adjust to the strategy you chose. With this in mind, setting a high expectation of exercise into your IF lifestyle may prove difficult to maintain to begin with. Keep in mind what we discussed around setting 'realistic' goals. There is no hard and fast rule to how much exercise you need to do so if you need to start small, do so. Some exercise is most definitely better than nothing. Similar to your IF plan you want to make sure your targets are safe and realistic to achieve. Exercising for 10 minutes every few days will dramatically accelerate your results without exhausting you. Every type of IF plan is adjustable enough to flex up or down in intensity and the same mindset can be applied to your exercise routine. Start with taking some long walks during the week and gradually increase the intensity by adding more activity based plans during your schedule.

Generally speaking, the more you exercise, the more benefit you get. The dual effect of exercising while IF is you will burn even more calories as your body uses stored fats for energy and your muscles are being put into action and will strengthen. A win win!

Pros and Cons of Exercising While Fasting

Exercising has its own great benefits. When combined with fasting, it produces more results. While there are enticing benefits to it, there are some cons to it as well. Let's begin with the pros.

It increases fat burning

Fasting and exercise can help burn more fat compared to exercising alone. This is because when you are exercising, the body burns the nutrients available at first, especially when you exercise not too long after eating a meal. After the body is done burning the nutrients while you are exercising, it starts burning stored fats in the body for energy.

It may help you lose stubborn fat.

One way or the other, everyone struggles with stubborn fats. They just vary in individuals based on genetics and different factors. How are they different? They differ in the alpha: beta ratio in the receptors contained in the fat cells and the blood flow the fat cells receive. The alpha receptors in the fat cells help reduce fat burning, while the beta receptors help encourage fat burning in the body. So, if the ratio favors the alpha receptors, it makes it harder for you to shed the stubborn fat in your body. The areas in your body where stubborn fat resides but receives less blood flow make it harder for you to burn the fat in that area because the fat-burning hormones won't be able to get to the fat in the area.

Fasting and exercising help increase the blood flow to the abdominal area where the most stubborn fat resides for everyone. So, combining both will help burn the stubborn fat in that area.

It helps you avoid an upset stomach.

Exercising with a full stomach can make you feel uncomfortable throughout your exercise. You can end up with an upset stomach. It can also result in indigestion, nausea, lethargy, etc. It can also slow down your training intensity. So, fasting while exercising helps you have a more comfortable and productive training exercise.

Cons of combining exercising and fasting

The following are the cons of exercising while fasting:

Decreased exercising intensity

People think you feel energetic in the morning and it is the right time for them to exercise. They haven't had breakfast yet, so they don't feel heavy. They are able to exercise for as long as they can. While this is true for some people, it is not the same for everyone. Some people feel weak and cannot exercise on an empty stomach. If they do, it slows them down, makes them weak and tired, and they are unable to be productive while exercising. That way, they can't get their desired results. When you don't have enough glucose *(which can be consumed through specific food or supplements prior to working out)* in your bloodstream, then your body would have to tap into the glycogen in your muscle. When that has been used, your body starts using up the fat in your body. However, it cannot break down fat as quickly as it breaks down the carbohydrate in your body. This makes you feel weak.

It increases your cortisol levels

Cortisol is the stress hormone in your body. Your body releases cortisol during times when it perceives threats. If you exercise intensely while you are fasting, you are likely to increase your cortisol level, leaving you stressed after the exercise. It could also prolong your raised cortisol levels. And high cortisol levels can stunt the fat-burning process and promote fat storage in your body. So, it's best you don't exercise intensely while you are fasting if you find that when you do you end up feeling more stressed than anything else, or you don't combine it at all. If you notice that your stress shoots up when you do both, it is best you refrain from doing that.

Exercising After a Meal

When you should exercise after a meal

It takes up to 2 to 4 hours for the food you eat to move to your small intestine. The food is slowly processed and goes into your small intestine little by little. It is not compulsory for you to wait till your food has digested before you start exercising. However, it is best if you let some time pass so the food can settle in your stomach. You can wait for 1 or 2 hours for regular size meals to settle and maybe 30 minutes for snacks to settle in your stomach. When you allow the food to digest enough, you can go ahead and exercise without worrying about an upset stomach. However, you should know that the more intense the exercise is, the higher your chance of experiencing some side effects.

Digestive discomforts

You may experience some digestive discomforts if you eat too much before you exercise. You may experience bloating, nausea, sluggishness, reflux, cramping, etc. You can avoid these side effects if you let your meal digest before you exercise.

It may affect your performance

Eating too close to your exercise can affect your performance. It makes you full and can result in sluggishness. When you feel this way, you won't be able to exercise as much as you ought to. You can experience nausea and keep belching throughout your exercising session. If you want to get the best result out of your exercising, it is best you don't eat at all, or you don't eat too much.

How long should you wait for each exercise?

Some exercises last a long time, so you might need to eat before you start. For example, swimming, cycling, and running require a lot of energy and may last a longer time than other exercises. So, you should eat high-digesting carbs before you start exercising. If you are running, you should wait 30 minutes after having a snack and between 1.5 to 3 hours after a meal. For walking, you can start after minimal time, whether you ate a snack or a heavy meal. For weight training, you should wait 30 minutes after a snack and 1 to 2 hours for a meal. Before you swim, you can wait 30 minutes after a snack and 1.5 to 3 hours after a meal.

Strength Training Exercises to Try at Home

Now we will look at some exercises you can do at home. The gym can be pretty intimidating if you are not used to the environment. Relying on the gym to be your base for exercise gives many of us the chance to make excuses for why we can't get there, the cost of the membership being daylight robbery and many other reasons causing exercise to take a back seat. With these easy at home exercises, there are no excuses not to give 20 minutes of your time to make a huge difference in the comfort of your own home.

- **The Plank**

The plank exercise will help you strengthen and tone your muscles. That is, it strengthens your abdominal and lowers back muscles. It also helps you to improve your balance. At the same time, it helps you to strengthen your posture. If you sit or stand all day or for most of your day, plank exercise will help you improve and maintain your posture throughout the day.

You can try the plank pose in different ways. You can try high plank or low plank. For the high plank, get in position, like when you do a push-up pose. Maintain straight arms and legs. You can try the low plank if you are a beginner. So, instead of keeping your arms straight, you can bend your arms at the elbow. So, you support your weight with your elbows. Whether you are trying the low or high plank, ensure that you maintain a straight posture, with your back straight and your head up. Your body should be like a parallel line to the floor.

- **Squats with chair**

You can also try squatting over a chair as another exercise. For this exercise, you squat over a chair in an almost sitting position. However, you don't sit on the chair. You don't make contact with the chair, and you stand right back up before you do. You then repeat this process a few more times. Squatting doesn't help you tone your lower body; however, it helps to strengthen your posture. You can start this exercise process by stretching your arms out in front of you as you squat. When you get better at it, you may choose not to.

- **Dumbbell floor press**

This is a weightlifting exercise that will help strengthen your chest muscles, arms and protect your shoulders. Women have weaker and underdeveloped chest muscles than men, so you can strengthen yours with this exercise. For this exercise, you need mats and dumbbells that you can lift. If you do not have a suitable bench, lie on the mat or floor if you like. Bend your knees and keep your feet flat on the floor. Take two dumbbells in your hands, one in one hand each. You then raise your arms over your chest. Lower your arms slowly to your side. Lower your arms and wrists, but don't let them touch the floor. Slightly bend your elbows, so you don't lock out your arms. Keep repeating this process a few more times.

- **Yoga**

You can also try out yoga. If you are an experienced yogi, you should know that there are different yoga styles that you can try. Some are somewhat strenuous, while some are easier. If you are trying out yoga for the first time, it is best you stay with the easy ones and not over-expand your strength. Focus more and stretch and balance for building your strength and muscle. You can try different poses on your chair or on the floor.

- **Modified push-up**

For this exercise, you need to get in a kneeling position on a mat. You need to arch your back and ensure that your legs are stretched on the mat. Then, place your palm on the mat. You would be in a push-up position, just that your knees would be touching the mat.

Tuck your toes under, tighten your abdominals, then bend your elbows to your lower chest towards the floor. Keep your eyes straight and let them focus on looking at your fingertips. Press your chest back up to the starting position. The targets for this exercise are your shoulders, arm, and core.

- **Stability ball tricep kickback**

For this exercise, hold dumbbells in your arms and place your chest on the ball. Let your arms drape beside the ball and stretch your legs out to the floor behind you. Let your head be straight in line with your spine. In case you don't have a ball to exercise with, you can lay your belly on a bench. After you have gotten into position, start by pulling your elbows up till they reach 90-degree angle. Pull your hands to the back to strengthen them, thereby squeezing your triceps. Release your arms to the starting position.

- **Shoulder overhead press**

First, you need to stand with your feet apart. Let your elbows down to your side while creating a space like a goalpost between them and your arms. Hold the dumbbells to the side of your head while you tighten your abdominals. Press dumbbells together over your head until your arms are straight. Then return your arms to the starting position. Repeat this a couple more times. You can also choose to sit while doing this exercise or on a stability ball while you keep your feet wide apart.

- **Stability ball overhead pull**

Rest your shoulder blades and head on the stability ball while the rest of your body forms a tabletop position. Keep your feet at a hip-distance apart from each other. Hold the dumbbells in your arms and hold them close to your chest. Raise the dumbbells together above your chest till your hands are straight. Let your palms face in rather than out as you raise them up. Then, slowly lower your arms to the back of your head and slightly bend your elbow. Pull your hands back to your chest, that is, the starting position. Squeeze your lats as you do this.

- **Stability ball side leg lift**

Get in a kneeling position with the ball on your right. Lean slightly on the ball and wrap your right arm around the ball. Extend your left leg while your right leg remains bent on the floor. Lift and lower your left leg slowly 8 to 12 times before you switch the ball to the other side. Repeat the same for the other side.

- **Bird dog**

Get on your knees on all fours. Raise one arm and stretch it out in front of you, draw in your abdominals and raise the opposite leg and stretch it out behind you. Put them back in position, and repeat 8 to 12 times. After you are done, switch arms and legs and repeat the same process for them.

Online Video Resources You Can Use For Your Exercise

Exercising is good for your body and health. So, here are some resources from YouTube you can use to stretch your bones and muscles when you need to exercise:

- Joe Wick's workout for seniors. The duration is 10 minutes, and you don't need any equipment for it.

- Joe Wick's 10-minute chair workout for seniors. You only need a chair and a can of food.

- Indoor walking workout- No equipment needed at all!

- Strength training for women over 50 You need two hand weights, dumbbells, or water bottles.

- High interval training (workout) for women over 50

Exercises are good for you. When combined with fasting, you get accelerated results. Combining exercise and fasting has its benefits. It helps you to lose weight and stubborn fats, improves your mental health, strengthens your bones, builds up your muscles, etc. This chapter has also provided some exercises you can try at home, as well as the description of videos that are tailored for over fifties that I encourage you to try!

Chapter Five:

Recipe for Different Goals While Fasting

The ultimate goal for most women reading this may be to lose stubborn weight, but there may be other elements of your health that you have always wanted to improve but just didn't know how to. Maybe you always feel tired and have a lack of energy to take on things that used to come so easily to you. Blood pressure may be a concern, but you've never had easy and tasty recipes to enjoy and lower your blood pressure at the same time. Here you will find recipes that lower your cholesterol, inflammation, strengthen bone density and so many more tailored recipes that can help with some of the 'secondary' goals you want to achieve.

Intermittent fasting in and of itself provides an amazing foundation for wonderful things to happen to your body and mind. This lifestyle enables you to have a regulated eating window and that is where the fun begins. As we explored in previous chapters, there is a control and power that scheduled eating provides. Knowing that there is a window for you to eat, should give you the motivation to plan ahead. By doing so, the recipes in this chapter will not only give you the ingredients and instructions on how to target your metabolism for instance, but healthy meals you can try and enjoy. You will also have the confidence in knowing they are accelerating you towards your goals and not slowing you down like some of the foods that may appear healthy but in reality are doing more damage than good.

Energizing Meals to Boost Your Day

Here are a few popular food choices known for being healthy and boosting energy. Perfect if you feel sluggish during your IF schedule and you need something to give you that bursts of energy you need.

Beef Liver

Beef liver is a great source for B12. Vitamin B12 helps prevent megaloblastic anemia, a blood condition that makes people tired and weak. This meal also contains loads of protein to keep you fueled and energised.

Oatmeal

Oatmeal is a simple and readily available food that is simple and quick to make. Adding a dash of honey or sweetener options would be a great way to make it more palatable if oatmeal is not a meal you regularly have. Oatmeal takes longer to digest than most meals, distributing energy evenly keeping you going for hours after you consume it. Stacked with nutrients and fibre, this is a fantastic option.

Beans

A fantastic source of protein with plenty of fibre to slow digestion, rich in magnesium which all helps your cells make energy. Probably not the 'sexiest' suggestion, sometimes healthy options don't have the zest you would expect however the benefits are undeniable.

Walnuts

Rich in omega-3 and walnuts in particular have one that your body uses for energy called 'alpha-linolenic' acid. Although walnuts (and nuts in general) are high in calories, studies have shown that those that consume high volumes of nuts do not gain weight.

Berries

An amazing substitute for refined sugar. The entire berrie family has natural sugars that will help boost your energy and provide antioxidants and other beneficial compounds that help nourish and protect the cells within your body.

Foods the Diabetic Should Eat Daily

People who are diabetic can still live a healthy life if only they can start eating right. Some unhealthy foods increase the blood sugar in the body and consequently cause type 2 diabetes. It has been discovered that some foods help diabetics to live better and also reduce the risk of having diabetes.

Blueberries

Researchers have discovered that frequent consumption of blueberries helps to boost the sensitivity of insulin. In other words, the body cell becomes open to insulin. There are several phytochemicals present in blueberries. These phytochemicals contain some anti-inflammatory substances. Therefore, the risk of having cardiovascular diseases and type 2 diabetes is drastically cut down.

Oranges

Citrus fruits such as oranges and grapefruits have a significant effect on the body's blood sugar. It also affects the cholesterol level of the body as well. It has been discovered that citrus fruits have hesperidin. This hesperidin is an anti-inflammatory compound that helps the body reduce the risk of having type 2 diabetes.

Chickpeas

Some foods have a low glycemic index. This makes them very important foods for diabetics. It has been discovered that diabetics who consume a significant quantity of legumes daily for twelve weeks experience improved health and a decreased effect of type 2 diabetes.

Vegetables

One of those people who have a very low risk of having type 2 diabetes is vegetarians. A diet that consists mainly of legumes, fruits and vegetables are one of the best and most recommendable therapeutic diets for persons suffering from type 2 diabetes. Research has shown that the blood glucose level can be reduced to about sixty-two per cent by taking a diet of vegetables, fruits and legumes.

Olive oil

The types of fats you consume affect your risk of worsening type 2 diabetes. Unsaturated fats are healthier than saturated and trans fats. This is because type 2 diabetes is closely associated with cardiovascular diseases and stroke. As much as possible, to maintain a healthy blood sugar level, you need to consume only heart-healthy fats.

Green vegetables

Type 2 diabetes has been discovered to experience the therapeutic effect in green vegetables. This is because green vegetables have vitamins A, vitamin C and Vitamin E and magnesium. These vitamins and elements have a low glycemic index.

Probiotics

Some bacteria have the ability to regulate the glucose and blood sugar levels in the body. One of the most popular foods that are high in probiotics is yoghurt. When consumed regularly, it has a significant impact on the blood sugar level.

Cinnamon

Cinnamon has been shown to increase the sensitivity of insulin in the body. Consequently, it is useful in maintaining a healthy sugar level in the body. It is a sweet spice that has been medically proven to have a strong therapeutic effect on the body glucose.

Healthy Evening Snacks Less Than 200 Calories

Are snacks entirely unhealthy for the body? There are times when you will crave something delicious and quick to eat. These cravings usually occur in the evenings. While eating very late has been discovered to make you gain weight, there are some snacks that have been discovered to even improve sleep. This is because they have certain compounds in them.

Tart cherries

Tart cherries have been discovered to aid better sleep. They also have anti-inflammatory compounds in them. They help to reduce your risk of developing several cardiovascular diseases and arthritis. If you are suffering from insomnia, try drinking a cup of cherry juice. Phytochemical procyanidin B-2 are present in tart cherries. More so, there are about 140 calories present in ⅓ of dry tart cherries.

Banana with almond butter

A combination of a small banana and about sixteen grams of almond butter has about 165 calories in it. This is a healthy snack that you can have in the evening when hunger pangs strike. It has also been proven to help improve better sleep. It helps to increase melatonin and serotonin in the body. Almonds have magnesium which is connected with good sleep.

Kiwi

Two peeled kiwis contain only ninety-three calories. It has also been proven to help improve better sleep. In case you are having difficulties with sleeping, kiwi is a go-to snack. This is because they contain a significant quantity of serotonin. Serotonin is a nerve messenger in the body. It helps to boost sleep performance as well as reduce your cravings for excessive carbs.

Pistachios

One unique characteristic that makes pistachios a healthy snack among other nuts is the presence of melatonin in it. This melatonin helps to improve sleep performance. It contains about one hundred and sixty calories.

Protein smoothie

Not only does a protein smoothie aid the repair of your muscle, but it also reduces the tendency of experiencing muscle loss. It is a delicious, easy-to-make and healthy snack for an evening. It has about one hundred and sixty calories. It also has tryptophan which aids the production or secretion of serotonin and melatonin.

Goji berries

Goji berries have a lot of carotenoids and antioxidants. A considerable amount of melatonin is also present in goji berries. This has a significant impact on overall sleep performance. You can eat them raw or mix them in a bowl of cereal.

Cheese and crackers

No other snack has a healthy combination of protein or carbohydrate like cheese and crackers do. This healthy snack helps to maintain a healthy level of sugar in the blood. Cheese has a tryptophan compound in it. Tryptophan consequently produces melatonin and serotonin, which boost sleep performance. While cheese has some great benefits, don't overdo it!

Filling Recipes for Meals Less Than 400 Calories Cooked in 20 Minutes

Seared scallops with chile-garlic spinach

It takes about twenty minutes to prepare. Some of the ingredients required include; cooking spray, kosher salt, ground black pepper, brown rice, olive oil, red onion, red Fresno chiles, garlic, spinach, and lemon wedges.

Nutritional information

- Calories - 368
- Fat – 7g
- Saturated fat – 1g
- Unsaturated fat – 6g
- Protein – 28g
- Carbohydrate – 50g
- Fibre – 7g
- Sugars – 3g
- Added sugar- 0g
- Sodium - 617mg
- Calcium - 14% DV
- Potassium – 14% DV

Steps to prepare it

1. Heat a skillet
2. Use the cooking spray coat pan
3. Sprinkle the scallops with salt and pepper
4. Add the scallops to the pan and cook for two minutes
5. Heat the rice and add the oil to a pan
6. Add onions, garlic, spinach and chiles in batches
7. Stir and cook for two minutes

Pan-seared shrimp with walnut and gremolata

It takes about fifteen minutes to prepare. The combination of shrimps, lemon and fresh herbs make this meal sumptuous. It is rich in proteins and has a small number of calories. Some of the ingredients needed to prepare Pan-seared shrimp with walnut and gremolata are; parsley, cilantro, garlic, walnuts, lemon, kosher salt, red pepper, olive oil, shrimps and spinach.

Nutritional information

- Calories - 401
- Fat – 20g
- Saturated fat – 3g
- Unsaturated fat – 16g
- Protein – 27g
- Carbohydrate – 26g
- Fibre – 3g
- Sugars – 1g
- Added sugar-   0g
- Sodium - 781mg
- Calcium - 17% DV
- Potassium – 11% DV

Steps to prepare it

1. Put the walnut, garlic, rind, salt, red pepper, cilantro, oil and parsley in a bowl and stir.
2. Heat the skillet
3. Cook the shrimps for about three minutes
4. Remove the shrimp and heat
5. Cook the garlic for about thirty seconds
6. Cook the spinach for about two minutes
7. Cook the brown rice pilaf for about one minute

Healthy Recipes To Lower High Blood Pressure

Vegan Superfood Grain Bowls

It is a delicious and healthy meal that can be prepared in fifteen minutes. It is dairy-free, egg-free, gluten-free, soy-free, nut-free. It is high in fibre and low in sodium and calories. Some of the ingredients include; quinoa, hummus, lemon juice, kale, edamame, avocado and sunflower seeds.

Nutritional values

- Serving size: 1 container
- Per Serving: 381 calories
- Protein: 16.2g
- Carbohydrates: 43.1g
- Dietary fibre: 13.2g
- Sugars: 7.7g
- Fat: 18.6g
- Saturated fat: 2.4g

Steps to prepare it

1. Cook the quinoa and allow it to cool
2. Mix the lemon juice and hummus in a bowl. Sprinkle with water and refrigerate
3. Sprinkle the quinoa, beets and edamame with sunflower seeds
4. Add the avocado to the mixture

Green Juice

This drink contains ingredients that help to reduce blood pressure naturally. Besides, part of the helpful tips includes losing excess body weight, eating plenty of plant foods, and aid daily body exercise. Remember, the smallest weight loss can have a significant influence on blood pressure. Ingredients for making the juice includes the following;

- 2 cucumbers
- 1 lemon

- Large bunch of parsley
- 4 celery sticks
- 1 green apple
- A knob of ginger (1 inch)

Directions

- Peel your lemon
- Chop and prepare produce to suit your juicer
- Sit and sip your juice

Magic Blood Pressure Reducer Juice

This type of vegetable juice recipe contains nitrate-rich veggies and anti-inflammatory ingredients. It is an effective blood pressure reducer, which tastes like a bloody Mary but without the vodka. The ingredients for making this juice include the following;

- 1 tablespoon beetroot powder
- ½ tomato juice low sodium
- ¼ cup carrot juice low sodium
- ¼ glass of water
- 1/8 teaspoon celery seed
- Teaspoon celery seed (1/8)
- 1/8 Teaspoon ginger (dried or minced)
- ice
- 1-ounce lime juice (1/2 lime)

Directions

- Get the beetroot powder and mix it with water. Ensure you measure the quantity and mix well.

- Add the tomato, Worcestershire sauce, carrot juice, celery seed, and ginger. Ensure you mix them very well.
- Add the lime juice, add the ice, and serve.

Anti-Aging Recipes

1. Paleo Sour Gummies

It contains an anti-inflammatory compound. It also boosts sleep performance. It helps to reduce joint pain. It also helps to keep a healthy body weight. Some of the ingredients include; lime, salt, orange and lemon.

Steps on how to prepare

1. Peel the lemons and oranges
2. Add lime and salt and blend for about two minutes
3. Put the mixture in a pot, add gelatin and stir well
4. Heat until the gelatin melts
5. Blend all the mixture again for about thirty seconds
6. Refrigerate before consuming

Nutritional information

- Calories: 73
- Carbs: 15g
- Sugar: 12g
- Protein: 2g

Cauliflower Mac 'n' Cheese

This baked mac and cheese contains carrots and cauliflower in the cheese sauce, making it a wholesome and healthy meal with all the elements needed to reduce the effects aging has on your body.. The ingredients for making this sumptuous meal include;

- Head cauliflower (1 piece)
- Medium carrots (4)
- 1 c. unsalted vegetable broth
- Teaspoon of salt (1/2)
- 1 pinch cayenne pepper (ground red)
- Teaspoon Dijon mustard (1)
- Teaspoon pepper (1/2)
- 12 oz. elbow macaroni ¼ c. parmesan cheese
- Medium plum tomatoes (2)
- ¾ c. Gruyere cheese
- 8 oz. small broccoli florets

Directions

1. First, you preheat to about 400 degrees F. Heat an 8-quart saucepan of salted water to a high boil.
2. Add carrots and cauliflower to boiling water for 15 minutes
3. In a blender, mix the cream cheese, mustard, black pepper, Gruyere, salt, cayenne, and broth. With your slotted spoon, add the veggies to the blender, and puree until tender.
4. Add your pasta to the pot of boiling water. Cook half-away and add broccoli. Stir in cauliflower sauce and half of your tomatoes.
5. Bake for 37 minutes or until the brown is on top and heated through

Spaghetti with Pesto Verde

This meal is a traditional pesto sauce that contains added flavour and vitamins for weight loss. Pesto may be high in calories due to containing olive oil nuts and cheese, the fats are primarily unsaturated. Pesto is full of antioxidants that help protect your cells from damage. The ingredients for this meal include the following;

- 1 clove of garlic
- 6 oz. baby spinach
- 10 oz frozen broccoli florets
- Teaspoon of fresh lemon juice
- Salt
- 1 c. fresh basil leaves
- 2 medium tomatoes
- 2 medium zucchini
- 2 teaspoon pine nuts

Directions

1. Heat a pot of salted water to a high point
2. In a microwave-safe bowl, mix your garlic, broccoli and add one cup of water.
3. Add your veggies peeler, peel zucchini into wide ribbons. And chop your tomatoes.
4. Cook spaghetti
5. Place cooled broccoli mixture, add your pine nuts, basil, lemon juice, black pepper, and ¼ teaspoon.
6. With a processor running, drizzle in oil. Add Parmesan and wait till it is well mixed.
7. Drain spaghetti well and return to the pot. Add your pesto, tomatoes, zucchini, and ¼ teaspoon salt and toss well.
8. Serve and eat well.

Improving Your Brain and Memory with Food

The brain is one of the major body organs in the body. It controls major body activities such as breathing, movement and heart beating. This is why it is very important to always ensure that the brain is as healthy as the body. The type of food you eat affects the functioning of the brain. Food can improve memory, concentration as well as the general mental wellbeing of the body.

1. Fish

Approximately sixty per cent of the brain is fat. About fifty per cent of this fat is made up of omega-3 fatty acids. This is why fatty fish is very good for the brain. Examples of fatty fishes are sardines, salmon, herring, albacore tuna and trout. These fishes contain omega-3 fatty acids. This omega-3 fatty acid helps in brain building. It is also very important for improved learning and brain memory. They also decrease the risk of Alzheimer's disease, depression and other learning impairments in the body. It has been discovered that persons who consume fish frequently are more likely to have a better brain than those who do not. This is because they have more grey matter in their brains. This grey matter is responsible for decision making, emotion and memory.

2. Coffee

Coffee contains antioxidants and caffeine. These two components are very important to maintain a healthy and improved brain. Caffeine helps to make the body more alert, although for the short term. This is because whenever coffee is taken into the body, a chemical messenger called adenosine is blocked. Adenosine is responsible for sleep. This way, the body stays alert as long as the caffeine is active in your system. It also helps the body to secrete dopamine hormone, also known as the feel-good hormone. When you drink coffee for a long time, you reduce the risk of having Alzheimer's disease as well as Parkinson's disease.

3. Turmeric

Turmeric is one of the healthy spicy foods that are good for the brain. It has an active ingredient called curcumin. Turmeric has a very high level of anti-inflammatory and antioxidants. For persons who may be suffering from Alzheimer's disease, curcumin works to improve the memory of the brain. It also improves mood by inducing the secretion of dopamine and serotonin. This way, it helps to fight anxiety and depression. It also helps new brain cells in the body to grow and develop.

4. Pumpkin seeds

Antioxidants present in pumpkin seeds help to protect the brain from damage. It also contains vital body compounds such as copper, iron, magnesium and zinc. Zinc and copper are important for nerve signaling. Magnesium helps improve memory and learning. Iron helps to prevent and fight impaired brain function such as brain fog. Generally, these compounds help to protect the body from Alzheimer's disease, Parkinson's disease, depression, migraine, epilepsy and other neurological conditions.

5. Chocolate

Generally, cocoa and chocolates contain antioxidants, caffeine and flavonoids for proper brain functioning. While regular milk chocolate has about ten to fifty per cent of cocoa, dark chocolate has about seventy percent of cocoa. Flavonoids are more active in the brain, where they help to improve learning and memory. Chocolate also helps to boost mood. Most milk chocolate has refined sugar and is high in calories, be careful not to over indulge.

Foods That Reduce Inflammation

The food you eat does not only contribute to your countenance, weight or energy; it affects how the body reacts and responds to ailments, inflammations and other body conditions. One of the ways the human body responds to immunity and fights infection is through inflammation. Whenever an inflammation in any part of the body becomes very severe, it can have a significant negative impact on the blood vessels, organs and joints. Different foods consequently cause different degrees of inflammation.

You need to know and understand how your body works so as to know which pro-inflammatory food that you should cut down on. Pro-inflammatory food may include; refined sugars and refined grains, white rice, potatoes, white bread, pastries, chips, refined crackers, pretzels and wheat. Some of these refined foods also cause high blood sugar. Baked foods, margarine and fried foods cause body inflammation. They clog the body's arteries and other blood vessels. To reduce inflammation in your body, you must cut down on red meat, processed meat, yoghurt, ice cream, cheese and butter. They contain saturated fats that not only make you at risk of heart disease but also increase inflammation in the body. On the contrary, anti-inflammatory foods will help you reduce the level of inflammation in your body. Some of these foods include:

1. Fiber

To reduce inflammation in your body, you need to consume a lot of fibre. Foods that are high in fibre include dark green vegetables, nuts, legumes, strawberries, pears and apples. These fibres not only help to reduce inflammation in the body, they also help to lose body weight.

2. Omega 3s

Omegas contain polyunsaturated fats that are good for the body and general physical wellbeing. Generally, they are found in fish. They help to reduce body inflammation. Foods that have polyunsaturated fats include sardines, salmon, tuna, rainbow trout and herrings. Researchers and dietitians have discovered that these fishes are best eaten as grilled, baked or boiled, and they must be eaten regularly.

3. Tomatoes and Dark Leafy Vegetables

Broccoli, eggplant, tomatoes, kale, collard, potatoes, spinach and peppers have been discovered to help reduce inflammation in the body. Nevertheless, they should be taken with great caution. Anyone suffering from some medical conditions such as arthritis may experience inflammation in the body if not taken with care.

4. Nuts

It has been discovered that antioxidants as well as vitamin E help the body to fight inflammation. They also help the body to repair worn-out tissue caused by inflammation and excessive activity in the immune system. Some popular nuts include; walnuts and almonds.

5. Olive oil

It has been discovered that olive oil has a compound called oleocanthal. This compound acts as a painkiller in the body. It helps the body to fight inflammation.

6. Berries and fruits

Raspberries, blueberries and strawberries have anti-inflammatory properties and antioxidants that help the body to stay healthy. Apples, oranges and tart cherries have been discovered to have a very high degree of the anti-inflammatory compound. They can be eaten raw or used to prepare salads.

7. Spices

If you are looking at eliminating or suppressing inflammation in your body, turmeric, oregano, ginger, cinnamon, parsley, and rosemary are the way to go. They have a high level of anti-inflammatory compounds to help keep your body healthy and hearty.

Low Cholesterol Recipes for a Healthier Heart

Gone are the days when low cholesterol diets used to be an option. It is no longer news that good health and cholesterol go hand in hand. Consuming high cholesterol puts you at risk of heart problems. Although cholesterol itself in the body is not entirely harmful, it is the connection of several heart diseases, and high cholesterol makes cholesterol a big issue. There are natural ways to help your body maintain a low cholesterol level. There are numerous low cholesterol recipes that you can make use of to help you live a healthier life. Can you do without cholesterol foods? That is almost impossible. This is because some foods naturally have good cholesterol in them that is healthy for the body. For example, sardines, eggs, yolk and cheese. Processed meat, fast foods and fried foods contain bad cholesterol that is not healthy for the heart. You must first understand that there are different types of cholesterol depending on the density of protein. HDL means High-Density Lipoprotein. LDL means Low-Density Lipoprotein. VLDL means Very Low-Density Lipoprotein. LDL and VLDL are bad cholesterol that is harmful to the body. HDL is the good cholesterol that is beneficial to the body. LDL and VLDL are capable of blocking the blood arteries and prevent blood from flowing to your heart. Some examples of low cholesterol recipes for a healthier heart include;

1. Low Cholesterol Meatloaf

Most times, many people think that to maintain a healthy cholesterol lifestyle, they have to do away totally with meat. This is not totally true. You do not have to feed on fruits and veggies regularly to maintain low cholesterol. With the low cholesterol meatloaf, you can enjoy your meat delicacies and still keep low cholesterol. One of the unique characteristics of the meatloaf is its ingredients. The ingredients used in making a meatloaf are mainly low in cholesterol. The ingredients are mainly fresh and natural rather than processed. Some of the ingredients include; carrots, oats and ground beef. These ingredients help to keep the heart healthy and reduce the risks of heart diseases. Carrot is rich in pectin. This makes it a very important vegetable in maintaining a healthy heart.

2. Chilled Avocado Soup

Have you ever had the avocado fruit blended into your dessert or salad? It is not only healthy but also very tasty and delicious. The avocado soup is best served chilled. It does not take much time to prepare as well. It has a mild taste and a great flavour. It is also very nutritious. It contains some healthy fats and vitamins. The avocado soup has monounsaturated fats. Some of the ingredients include spices, low-fat yoghurt and lemon.

3. Broccoli Almond

The broccoli Almond recipe is a delicious dish that is a healthy green vegetable for the heart. The recipe is made up of broccoli and almond nuts, chicken broth, butter and garlic. These ingredients make it a sumptuous dish that is low in cholesterol. The broccoli vegetable is rich in Vitamin A, B, C, E, K, protein, calcium, fibre and iron. It also contains some soluble fibre present in some grains. An almond nut is rich in potassium, calcium and magnesium that are generally important in maintaining a healthy heart. The broccoli almond recipe is simple and quick to prepare.

4. Bean Salad with Pine Nuts and Feta

If you are looking to cut down on bad cholesterol levels in your body, the bean salad with pine nuts and feta is one of the best dishes that you can take. The combination of feta cheese, beans and pine nuts is nutritious, tasty and delicious. Another recipe for this dish may include; parsley, honey, onions, cucumber, olives and bell peppers. The Bean Salad with Pine Nuts and Feta is simple and quick to prepare. Most legumes such as lentils, peas and beans have low cholesterol content, and they contain vitamins, fibre and protein. Nuts like walnuts, almonds and pine nuts are able to lower the level of cholesterol in the body. The feta cheese contains a high level of vitamin A, zinc, potassium, iron, vitamin B6 and phosphorus.

Chapter Six:

Breakfast, Lunch, and Snack Recipes

Pumpkin Powerhouse

Ingredients

- 1/2 frozen banana (adds creaminess and sweetness without added sugar)
- 1 cup pumpkin puree (canned or fresh)
- a handful of ice cubes
- 1 cup unsweetened vanilla almond milk
- dash of pumpkin pie spice (swap for cinnamon if you don't have this)

Blend all ingredients together.

Green Sunrise Smoothie

Ingredients:

- 1 scoop protein powder (Miller uses Medifast's Pineapple Mango Smoothie packet)
- 1 cup unsweetened almond or cashew milk
- 1 tablespoon ground flaxseed
- 1 cup fresh spinach
- 1½ oz sliced avocado

Blend all ingredients together

Chia-Berry Belly Blaster

Ingredients:

- 1 tablespoon ground chia seeds
- 1/2 cup ice
- 1 cup frozen berries (blueberries, strawberries, or açai berries make great options)
- 1 tablespoon vanilla extract
- 1 cup plain Greek yogurt, unsweetened
- Blend all ingredients together

Spicy Tropical Greens Delight

Ingredients:

- 1/4 tablespoon cayenne pepper (optional)
- 1 cup frozen pineapple chunks
- 1/4 cup lime juice
- 1 1/2 unsweetened coconut water
- 1 cup leafy greens (baby spinach, kale, collard greens, etc.)

- 1 cup frozen mango chunks

Blend all ingredients together. You can use this recipe for two servings.

Vanilla-Berry Blast

Ingredients:

- 1 quart plain nonfat Greek yogurt
- 1 tablespoon cinnamon
- 1 banana, frozen
- 8 ounces unsweetened frozen strawberries or blueberries
- 2 cups unsweetened vanilla almond milk

Add half of each of the yogurt, berries, and milk into a blender and blend until it is smooth. Add the remainder of the ingredients and blend until smooth. You can use this recipe for three servings. You can refrigerate or share with people in three glasses.

Spirulina Smoothie

Ingredients:

- 1 banana
- 1 tsp spirulina
- 1/2 cup coconut water
- 1 scoop vegan vanilla protein powder (optional)
- 1/2 cup almond milk

Blend all ingredients together.

Belly-Busting Berry Smoothie

Ingredients:

- 1 cup almond milk
- handful of ice
- 1 cup frozen berries (strawberries, raspberries, blackberries, etc.)
- 1 tbsp almond or peanut butter
- 1 banana

Blend all ingredients together.

Another major component in our daily intake is snacks. Most of the common snacks have high amounts of calories and would not be advisable for people trying to lose weight. However, there are some snacks that you can take that do not defeat the purpose of intermittent fasting. Below is a list that you can choose from;

Snacks Under 100 Calories

Simple Snacks under 100 Calories

Don't have a lot of time but are in need of a hunger fix? Here are some terrific go-to's, all under 100 calories.

1. 20 pistachios – 80 calories
2. 75g tin of tuna in spring water – 81 calories
3. one boiled egg – 70 calories
4. two cups of air-popped popcorn – 60 calories
5. 14 almonds – 98 calories

Sweet snacks under 100 Calories

These are perfect if you're a sweet tooth or if you have flown through a fast day with calories left for dessert!

1. two cups of watermelon – 90 calories
2. baked apple with cinnamon – 95 calories
3. 250 g punnet of strawberries – 80 calories
4. 2 tsp. of peanut butter and two stalks of celery – 68 calories
5. three squares of dark chocolate – 77 calories

Savory snacks under 100 Calories

These easy-peasy savory options prove you don't have to reinvent the wheel to go low-cal!

1. Rice or corn thin with sliced tomato and 1 tbsp. parmesan cheese – 53 calories
2. two cups carrot and celery sticks – 70 calories
3. two slices of crispbread, 1/2 teaspoon Vegemite & 1/2 teaspoon butter – 92 calories
4. one cup of miso soup – 35 calories
5. 1/4 medium avocado smashed with five cherry tomatoes, halved – 98 calories

Substantial snacks under 100 Calories

Looking for something a little more substantial without the calories? These light lunch or dinner options will satisfy your stomach.

1. One cup sliced strawberries, a quarter of a packet of baby spinach, 1 tbsp. balsamic vinegar – 56 calories
2. 100 g sweet potato steamed or baked with 1 tsp. curry powder – 94 calories

3. 50 g shredded chicken and 10 strips of capsicum – 90 calories
4. one cup tomatoes, one cup cucumber, ½ cup onion, five olives, and 1 tbsp. balsamic vinegar – 92 calories
5. two slices of turkey breast wrapped in a lettuce leaf – 60 calories

On The Go Snacks

Many times when you are trying to keep up with the busy nature of the modern world, you will not have time to prepare a meal, and on such occasions, snacks can be very useful when you are hungry. However, the majority of the snacks in the modern world are rich in refined carbs and sugar, which leaves you unsatisfied and increases your craving for food. The best snacks are those that are rich in protein and nutritious. Protein makes you more satisfied by its release of appetite-suppressing hormones. Proteinous foods are slowly digested and stabilize the level of your blood sugar. Here is a list of 30 protein snacks that are portable and healthy.

Jerky

Jerky is made from trimming the fat from meat, cut into parts, and dried. It is convenient and good as a snack. It is rich in protein as it contains about 9 grams per ounce. You can use beef, chicken, salmon, and turkey. You can get it in grocery stores, although jerky sold in grocery stores is usually high in added sugar and other artificial ingredients if you want the best jerky to make it yourself or go to a local butcher that will have it fresh for you.

Trail mix

Trail mix is a mixture of dried fruit and nuts that you can combine with chocolate and grains sometimes. Trail mix is an excellent source of protein as it provides 8 grams in a 2-ounce serving. The amount of protein in the trail mix is dependent on you; you can use almonds or pistachios instead of nuts as they have the highest protein content. It is rich in calories; you should eat it moderately.

Turkey roll-ups

Turkey roll-ups is a delicious and highly nutritious protein snack made up of cheese and veggies wrapped in slices of turkey breast. This protein snack is high in protein and low in carbohydrates. Studies have shown that it can improve blood sugar levels which is an important factor in appetite regulation.

Greek yogurt parfait

Greek yogurt is a healthy snack rich in protein. It contains about 20 grams of protein in every serving cup.

Veggies and yogurt dip

Veggies are a good option for snacks, but they do not have high protein content. You can increase the protein content by adding yogurt dip to it.

Tuna

Tuna is rich in protein, and this makes it a very convenient and healthy snack option. Each cup of tuna is loaded with about 39 grams of protein.

Hard-boiled eggs

Eggs are very healthy, and they contain all nutrients needed by the body. One boiled egg contains about 6 grams of protein, and you can use it as a snack.

Peanut butter celery sticks

Celery sticks that contain 1-2 tablespoons of peanut butter are delicious and can be used as a snack. Each tablespoon of peanut butter contains about 4 grams of protein.

No-bake energy bites

Energy bites are delicious, and they contain huge amounts of protein by combining various ingredients like oats, nut butter.

Cheese slices

Cheese is a very healthy, quick, and easy snack. Cheese slices are rich in protein, with each slice containing about 7 grams of protein. It is also incredibly filling. This is one that you need to be moderate with.

Handful of almonds

You can eat a handful of almonds or other types of nuts as a snack. They are rich in protein; one ounce of almonds contains about 6 grams of protein.

Roasted chickpeas

Chickpeas are a legume that has huge amounts of nutrients. Some of those nutrients are protein and fiber.

Hummus and veggies

Hummus is made from mashed and cooked chickpeas, which are blended with olive or tahini oil. They can be used as a spread, and 1/3 cup of hummus contains 4 grams of protein. You can eat it with vegetables as a snack.

Cottage cheese

Cottage snack is a filling snack that is known predominantly for its huge amounts of protein. Each half-cup contains about 14 grams of protein.

Apple with peanut butter

Not only does this go together, but they are also good sources of nutrients, especially protein, and provide some health benefits.

Protein bars

Protein bars make it easy for you to consume huge amounts of protein. Although it is better, you make them on your own as the store versions have been compromised with unnecessary ingredients.

Canned salmon

Canned salmon is a very good source of protein, and you can take it along anywhere. One ounce of canned salmon provides 8 grams of protein.

Chia pudding

Chia pudding is a very popular snack because it has high amounts of protein. It is also delicious and healthy.

Homemade granola

Granola contains rolled oats, nuts, and a sweetener like honey which are baked together. It is very filling because of its high protein content.

Pumpkin seeds

Pumpkin seeds are excellent options if you are looking for a quick snack. They are high in protein and other essential nutrients.

Nut butter

You can find this portable and quick high-protein snack in grocery stores. They are rich in nutrients and provide huge amounts of fats, vitamins B, magnesium, phosphorus, and Vitamin E.

Protein shakes

Although you can get protein from food, protein shakes are also excellent sources of protein that can be used as a snack.

Edamame

Edamame beans are a kind of soybeans that are immature and still in the pod. They are rich sources of protein, minerals, and vitamins that can be used as an easy snack.

Avocado and chicken salad

You can use avocado and chicken salad as a portable and filling snack. The mixture of protein from chicken and healthy fats will make you full and satisfied.

Fruits and nut bars

You can use fruits and nut bars as a portable snack that is rich in protein.

Lentil salad

You can consume the lentil salad as a great snack. The lentil salad is rich in nutrients, and it is a good plant-based source of protein.

Overnight oatmeal

It is easy to make overnight oatmeal, and it is highly nutritious and portable. Oats are high in protein, and they are filled with huge amounts of vitamins and minerals.

Brunch Recipes

Scrambled Egg with Sweet Potatoes

Ingredients:

- 1 (8-oz) sweet potato, diced
- 2 tablespoons chopped chive
- ½ cup chopped onion
- 4 large egg whites
- Salt
- Pepper
- 2 tablespoons chopped rosemary
- 4 large eggs

Directions:

1. Preheat the oven to 246° C. On the baking sheet, toss the sweet potato, onion, rosemary, and salt, and pepper. Spray with cooking spray and keep roasting till it is tender for about 20 minutes.
2. Also, in a medium bowl, whisk together the eggs, egg whites, and a pinch of salt and pepper. Spray a skillet with cooking spray, and you scramble the eggs on medium for about 5 minutes.
3. Sprinkle the mixture with chopped chives and serve with spuds.

Ensure that each serving does not exceed 571 calories, 44 g protein, 52 g carbs, and 20 g fat.

Greek Chickpea Waffles

Ingredients:

- Salt and pepper
- ¾ cup chickpea flour
- 6 large eggs
- ¾ cup plain 2% Greek yogurt
- Tomatoes, parsley, cucumbers, yogurt, scallion, olive oil and lemon juice for serving (optional)
- ½ tsp salt
- ½ tsp baking soda

Directions:

1. Start by preheating your oven to 93°C. Put a wire rack on top of your rimmed baking sheet and put it in the oven. Proceed to heat the waffle iron per direction.

2. Mix the baking soda, flour, and salt in a large container. You can make use of a small container to mix the yogurt and eggs. Mix the wet and dry ingredients.
3. Gently coat the waffle iron with a nonstick cooking spray. Add a quarter into half cup batter into each section of the iron and cook until you get a golden brown color, 4 to 5 minutes; you should do this in batches. Move the waffles to the oven and maintain it at a warm temperature. Repeat this process with the remaining batter.
4. Serve waffles with a savory tomato mix, or you can use a sprinkle of warm nut butter and berries.
5. The ingredients here are for two servings.

In every serving, there should be about 412 calories, 35 g protein, 24 g carbs, and 18 g fat present.

PB&J Overnight Oats

Ingredients:

- butter
- ¼ cup mashed raspberries
- ¼ cup quick-cooking rolled oats
- 3 tbsp creamy peanut
- ½ cup 2 percent milk
- 3 tbsp whole raspberries

Directions:

1. Mix oats, milk, peanut butter, and mashed raspberries in a medium bowl and Stir until smooth.
2. You should cover the mixture and refrigerate it overnight. In the morning, uncover and put toppings of raspberries.

You should have up to 455 calories, 20 g protein, 36 g carbs, and 28 g of fat.

Turmeric Tofu Scramble

Ingredients:

- 1 tbsp olive oil
- ½ block (14-oz) firm tofu
- 1 portobello mushroom
- ¼ tsp ground turmeric
- Pinch garlic powder
- 3 or 4 cherry tomatoes
- ½ avocado, thinly sliced
- Salt and pepper

Directions:

1. Start by preheating your oven to 204°C. Place the shroom and tomatoes on your baking sheet and brush them with oil. Add salt and pepper and roast for about 10 minutes till it is tender.
2. Meanwhile, mix the garlic powder, tofu, turmeric with a pinch of salt and mash the mixture with a fork. Using a large skillet at medium heat, heat a tablespoon of olive oil. Proceed to add the tofu mixture and cook. During the process of cooking, occasionally stir until it is firm and egg-like for about 3 minutes. Plate the tofu and serve with mushroom, avocado, and tomatoes.

You should have about 431 calories, 21 g protein, 17 g carbs, and 33 g fat in every serving.

Avocado Ricotta Power Toast

Ingredients:

- 1 slice whole-grain bread
- ¼ ripe avocado smashed
- 2 tbsp ricotta
- Pinch crushed red pepper flakes
- Pinch flaky sea salt

Directions:

1. Start by toasting the bread. Top with avocado, crushed red pepper flakes, ricotta, and sea salt. Eat with scrambled or hard-boiled eggs and a serving of yogurt or fruit.

Ensure that you have 288 calories, 10 g protein, 29 g carbs, and 17 g fat in each serving.

Turkish Egg Breakfast

Ingredients:

- ¾ cup diced red bell pepper
- ¼ tsp paprika
- 2 dollops plain yogurt
- 1 whole-wheat pita
- Chopped cilantro to taste
- ¾ cup diced eggplant
- Pinch each of salt and pepper
- 5 large eggs, lightly beaten
- 2 tablespoon olive oil

Directions:

1. In a large nonstick skillet with the temperature set at medium-high, heat the olive oil. Add the bell pepper, salt, and eggplant, and pepper. Sauté until softened, about 7 minutes.
2. Stir in the pepper, paprika, and more salt and eggs to taste. You should stir the dish often while cooking until the eggs are softly scrambled.
3. Sprinkle with chopped cilantro and serve with a dollop of yogurt and the pita.
4. Ingredients here are for two servings

Almond Apple Spice Muffins

Ingredients:

- ½ stick butter
- 2 cups almond meal
- 4 scoops of vanilla protein powder
- 4 large eggs
- 1 cup unsweetened applesauce
- 1 tbsp cinnamon
- 1 tsp allspice
- 1 tsp cloves
- 2 tsp baking powder

Directions:

1. Preheat your oven to 350° F. You should use a small microwave-safe bowl to melt the butter in the microwave on low heat, about 30 seconds.
2. You can use a large container to mix all the remaining ingredients thoroughly with melted butter. Spray 2 muffin

tins using a nonstick cooking spray, or you can use cupcake liners.

3. Transfer the mixture into muffin tins and make sure you do not overfill (about ¾ full). You should be able to make 10 muffins.

4. Put one tray in the oven and allow it to bake for about 12 minutes. Make sure you do not overbake them, as the muffins will become very dry. When the first tray is completely baked, remove it from the oven and bake the second muffin in the same manner.

Ensure that you have 484 calories, 40 g protein, 16 g carbs, and 31 g fat in all servings.

Dinner Recipes

Turkey Tacos

Ingredients:

- 1 cup chopped lettuce
- 1 clove garlic, finely chopped
- 1 tbsp sodium-free taco seasoning
- 2 tsp oil
- 8 whole-grain corn tortillas, warmed
- ¼ cup sour cream
- ½ cup shredded Mexican cheese
- 1 avocado, sliced
- Salsa, for serving
- 1 lb. extra-lean ground turkey
- 1 small red onion, chopped

Directions:

1. In a large skillet, set the temperature to medium-high and heat the oil. Add onion to the oil and cook; keep mixing until the mixture becomes tender. This process should take about 5 to 6 minutes. Add the garlic and cook for a minute.
2. Add the turkey into the mixture and cook; break it up with a spoon wait until it is nearly brown. This should take about 5 minutes. Pour in the taco seasoning with a cup of water. Simmer until it is reduced by more than half in seven minutes.
3. Fill the tortillas by using turkey and top it with lettuce, sour avocado cream, cheese, and salsa.

Healthy Spaghetti Bolognese

Ingredients:

- 1 large spaghetti squash
- ¼ lb. ground turkey
- 8 oz. small cremini mushrooms, sliced
- 1 (8-oz) can low-sodium, no-sugar-added tomato sauce
- ½ tsp garlic powder
- 3 cups fresh diced tomatoes
- 1 small onion, finely chopped
- 3 tbsp olive oil
- Kosher salt and pepper
- 4 cloves garlic, finely chopped
- Fresh chopped basil

Directions:

1. Preheat your oven to 204° C. Cut the spaghetti squash in half lengthwise and throw away the seeds. Rub each half

with 1/2 tablespoon oil and follow this by seasoning with garlic powder and ¼ tsp each salt and pepper. Ensure that the skin side is up on a rimmed baking sheet and roast until it is tender for about 35 to 40 minutes. Let it cool down for 10 minutes.

2. You should also heat the remaining 2 Tbsp oil in a large skillet on medium. Add the onion, season with a quarter of a tablespoon for salt and pepper and cook. Ensure that you occasionally stir until tender for about 6 minutes. Add the turkey by breaking it up into small pieces with a spoon and cook until it is browned for about 6 to 7 minutes. Mix it in the garlic and cook for a minute.

3. Push the turkey mixture to one side of the pan, and include the mushrooms in the other. Cook and occasionally stir until you have tender mushrooms in about 5 minutes. Pour the mixture into the turkey and follow this up by adding the tomatoes and tomato sauce and let it simmer for 10 minutes.

4. When the sauce is simmering, take a scoop out the squash and serve it. Spoon the turkey Bolognese over the top and sprinkle with basil based on your preference.

Chicken with Fried Cauliflower Rice

Ingredients:

- ½ cup frozen peas, thawed
- 4 large eggs, beaten
- 2 tbsp low-sodium soy sauce
- 4 scallions, finely chopped, plus more for serving
- 2 red bell peppers, finely chopped
- 2 tsp rice vinegar
- 2 tbsp grapeseed oil
- 2 small carrots, finely chopped

- 1 onion, finely chopped
- Kosher salt and pepper
- 1 ¼ lb. boneless, skinless chicken breast, pounded till thickness is even
- 2 cloves garlic, finely chopped
- 4 cups of cauliflower "rice."

Directions:

1. Heat 1 tbsp oil and a large, deep skillet at a temperature of medium-high. Add the chicken and cook until you get a golden brown color; it can be done for 3 to 4 minutes per side. Move it to a cutting board and allow it to rest for 6 minutes before cutting. Add remaining 1 tablespoon of oil to the skillet. Add the eggs and scramble until it is set after 1 to 2 minutes. Proceed to transfer into a bowl.
2. Add the bell pepper, carrot, and onion to the skillet and cook. You should often stir until it is tender after 4 or 5 minutes. Mix in the garlic and cook for a minute. Toss with peas and scallions.
3. Add the cauliflower, soy sauce, rice vinegar, salt, and pepper and mix by tossing. This should be followed by allowing the cauliflower to sit, without stirring, until beginning to brown, 2 to 3 minutes. Toss with the sliced chicken and eggs.

Sheet Pan Steak

Ingredients:

- 1 lb. small cremini mushrooms, trimmed and halved
- 1 ¼ lb. bunch broccolini, trimmed and cut into 2-in. lengths
- 3 tbsp olive oil

- 2 1-in.-thick New York strip steaks (about 1½ lb total), trimmed of excess fat
- 4 cloves garlic, finely chopped
- ¼ tsp red pepper flakes (or a bit more for extra kick)
- Kosher salt and pepper
- 1 15-oz can low-sodium cannellini beans, rinsed

Directions:

1. You should start by preheating the oven to 450° F. Toss the garlic, mushrooms, red pepper flakes, broccolini, oil, and quarter of a tablespoon of salt and pepper on your large rimmed baking sheet. Put the baking sheet in the oven and leave it to roast for 15 minutes.
2. Push the mixture to the pan edges to create room for the steaks. Season the steaks with a quarter of a tablespoon for salt and pepper and place in the middle of the pan. Roast your steaks to the desired degree for about 5 to 7 minutes on each side if you want medium-rare. Move the steaks to a cutting board and allow it to rest for 5 minutes before slicing.
3. Add beans to the baking sheet and mix by tossing. Roast until you have heated it completely for about 3 minutes. Serve the beans and vegetables with steak.

Pork Tenderloin with Butternut Squash and Brussels Sprouts

Ingredients:

- 1 ¾ lb. pork tenderloin, trimmed
- Salt
- 4 cups diced butternut squash

- Pepper
- 2 sprigs of fresh thyme
- 3 tbsp canola oil
- 2 garlic cloves, peeled
- 4 cups Brussels sprouts, trimmed and halved

Directions:

1. Start by preheating your oven to 400° F. Season the tenderloin throughout with salt and pepper. In a large cast-iron pan at medium-high temperature, heat 1 tablespoon of oil. When the oil shimmers, proceed to add the tenderloin and let it sear until you get a golden brown on all sides. This process should be completed in 8 to 12 minutes total. Transfer the tenderloin into a plate.

2. Add thyme and garlic and remaining two tablespoons of oil to the pan and cook until aromatic for about 1 minute. Add the butternut squash, a big pinch each of salt and pepper and Brussels sprouts. Occasionally stir the mixture when cooking until the vegetables are slightly browned in 4 to 6 minutes.

3. Place the tenderloin over the vegetables and transfer everything to the oven. Roast until the vegetables are tender and insert a meat thermometer into the thickest part of the tenderloin and keep roasting until you register 140°F. This should take 15 to 20 minutes.

4. Ensure you wear oven mitts to remove the pan from the oven carefully. Allow the tenderloin to rest for about 5 minutes before you slice and serve with the vegetables. Toss greens with a balsamic vinaigrette to serve as a side dish.

Wild Cajun Spiced Salmon

Ingredients:

- 3 tbsp olive oil
- 1½ lb. wild Alaskan salmon fillet
- ½ tsp garlic powder
- 1 head broccoli and cut into florets
- Sodium-free taco seasoning
- ½ head cauliflower (cut into florets
- 4 medium tomatoes, diced

Directions:

1. Preheat the oven to 375° F. Place the salmon in a baking dish. In a small bowl, mix the taco seasoning with ½ cup water. Pour the mixture over the salmon and bake until opaque throughout, 12 to 15 minutes.
2. Meanwhile, in a food processor (in batches as necessary), pulse the cauliflower and broccoli until finely chopped and "riced."
3. In a large skillet on medium, heat the oil. Add the cauliflower and broccoli, sprinkle with garlic powder, and cook, tossing until just tender, 5 to 6 minutes.
4. Serve salmon on top of "rice" and top with tomatoes.

Pork Chops with Bloody Mary Tomato Salad

Ingredients:

- ¼ cup finely chopped flat-leaf parsley
- 2 tbsp olive oil
- 2 tbsp red wine vinegar
- ½ tsp Tabasco

- 1 small head green-leaf lettuce, leaves torn
- 2 tsp Worcestershire sauce
- Kosher salt
- ½ tsp celery seeds
- 4 small bone-in pork chops (1 in. thick, about 2¼ lb total)
- Pepper
- 2 tsp prepared horseradish, squeezed dry
- 2 celery stalks, very thinly sliced
- 1-pint cherry tomatoes halved
- ½ small red onion, thinly sliced

Directions:

1. Heat your grill to a medium-high temperature. In a large container, whisk the oil together, Worcestershire sauce, horseradish, vinegar, Tabasco, celery seeds, and quarter of a tablespoon of salt. Toss with the celery, onion, and tomatoes.
2. Season the pork chops with ½ tablespoon of salt and pepper and grill until you get a golden brown and you cook through, 5 to 7 minutes on each side.
3. Fold the parsley into the tomatoes and serve with pork and greens. Eat with mashed cauliflower or potatoes.

Chapter Seven:

Combining Intermittent Fasting and The Keto Diet

Combining intermittent fasting and keto diet means eating more fats and restricting intake of carbs at some specific times of the day. Ordinarily, both intermittent fasting and the keto diet are used for the same purpose – there are panaceas for weight loss.

Reducing the carb intake and fueling the body with fats are what both intermittent fasting and keto dieting are all about. They are both effective ways to reduce weight and add more fats needed in the body for proper functioning. As a woman above fifty, adopting this combination without medical consultation is not advisable. However, it is important to know that many women have expressed some amazing results when combining the two methods together. Throughout this book you may have noticed multiple references to consulting your doctor and this is purely for your benefit. Sudden and drastic changes to the diet in most cases causes a positive reaction (if done in the right way). However, there is no harm in getting a medical opinion from a doctor who understands your medical history and the potential downsides to making this leap. This is not to say that some women will be strongly advised to avoid the keto diet and IF combination, it may be a case of taking a more considered and 'one step at a time' approach.

While thinking of adopting this method, it would be considered thoughtful and healthier to know about the combination of the two. Although scientifically, there has never been a study or research effort to validate the effectiveness of this approach for weight loss. Most people only think that the approach will likely produce effective results based on the two dieting methods' purpose. Likewise, experts say the combo can make sense, though the lack of research efforts in this area might want you to think twice before adopting the method.

Combining the diets gained popularity when Jason Fung, an intermittent fasting expert and the author of *The Obesity Code,* recommended the use of the Ketogenic diet as a foundation to IF. Dr. Lori Shemek, a nutritionist and weight loss expert, confirmed that he had recommended the approach to his patients.

At this junction, it is worthwhile to enhance your understanding of what the Ketogenic diet means. Remember, the concept of intermittent fasting has been thoroughly explained to you, most especially as it relates to your gender, age, and health goals. That's why it is a thought worth considering to talk a bit about the Keto diet.

Understanding the Basics of Keto Diet

According to previous research, the diet was primarily designed by scientists in the 1920s to help children struggling with epilepsy or seizures cases. The ketogenic diet version calls for eating 3 to 4 grams of fat for every 1 g of protein and carb. That information is according to the Epilepsy Foundation.

The version that many are using for weight loss nowadays is a bit different because the protein content is moderate, and it entails a low-carb and high-fat plan. The idea is to have the intake of daily calories at 80%. That implies you have to consume between 20 to 50 g of net carbs every day, depending on your health goals.

The normal keto diet food list requires ditching most carbs. It calls for eating healthy foods such as fruits and veggies. It also prioritizes eating foods such as olive oil, avocado, bacon, and grass-fed beef on rare occasions.

The plan with this eating method is to transit your body from one that burns glucose or carbs for fuel to gain energy. As a woman above fifty, the glucose or carbs you consume should be converted to energy that the body requires to function effectively. This process is called ketosis. If your body is keto-adapted, this method can be a good fit for you. This process is one of the effective ways or strategies to reduce weight in a very short time. Notwithstanding, critics reveal that long-term research on this method's effectiveness on people with weight loss cases is insufficient and lacking.

Why Has Combining Intermittent Fasting and Ketogenic Dieting Gained Popularity?

Combining the keto diet and IF can help produce weight loss in the short term. However, it is crucially important to note that each plan is very restrictive. They certainly are not for everyone. As a woman above fifty, you may need to study the restrictive tendencies alongside your doctor's prescription before deciding to adopt the method.

What do you really feel about combining them? Could the two be better?

First, we need to consider the experts' point of view. In some experts' perspectives, it really makes sense to combine the two. The keto diet increases the level of the ketones in the body; during fasting days, ketones are also released.

According to Dominic D'Agostino, Ph.D., associate professor at the University of South Florida in Tampa and founder of KetoNutrition, "The brain will rely less on glucose for energy when in a state of nutritional ketosis. Therefore, the transition into a fasted (ketogenic) state during the day eventually becomes seamless after eating low-carb or ketogenic for a few weeks."

The Right Way to Adopt This Approach

Now that you have read that the combination might really be healthful and helpful to achieving your weight loss goal, it is essential to understand the right way to adopt this approach to avoid the side effects.

As a woman above fifty, practitioners may not advise you to start both at the same time. For instance, practitioners at Cleveland Clinic do not advise their patients to start the intermittent fasting keto diet at the same time. "It's a huge shock to your system to switch from glucose as fuel to ketones, and implementing IF is a significant change," says Kwasnicka. For that reason, you may not be advised to start with keto. After you have been dieting for a couple of weeks, you can consider intermittent fasting.

That said, it is essential to choose the right timing. As women above fifty, you can consider a 10 to 12-hour fast. For most women at your age, not eating for 12 hours is a normal and natural habit.

And if you belong to this category, it does not take special effort rather than skipping meals.

For a start, you consider delaying your breakfast. This is necessary because your body needs to get accustomed to the new eating habit. It would get your body going on a long stretch without eating. When your body has been adjusted to the new eating pattern, then you can reintroduce your breakfast in the day and extend your eating time at night. Eating breakfast helps to increase your metabolism state and insulin sensitivity.

In sum, you have learned to combine intermittent fasting and the keto diet to achieve your weight loss. But one thing you may need to include is the time you need to stay on this approach. Experts advised that women above fifty are expected to be on intermittent keto fasting for six months and then change to a more standard low-carb diet. However, it is advisable to combine this method the right way to avoid any potential effects.

Chapter Eight:

FAQs and Answers About Intermittent Fasting

Having understood the need to combine the two approaches to achieve your weight loss goal faster and easier, you need to take a step further to look at some frequently asked questions on the concept of intermittent fasting, particularly as it concerns women above fifty years.

Many women who are interested in intermittent fasting have been asking pertinent questions about how healthy dieting is to people in their category. They want to know how healthy, reliable, and effective they are. This method is in achieving their health goals.

Many women above fifty who are interested in IF are asking these questions, and we can't hide away from that.

Let's get started with questions on how to start intermittent fasting.

Questions About How to Start Intermittent Fasting

Here, we will answer a few questions women over 50 asked about how to start intermittent fasting. We shall look at common mistakes that women make and how to get started properly.

Q: Can I have a fruit or two fruits (apple and banana) between meals? For example, the first meal at 1 pm, fruit at 4 pm, second meal at 8 pm.

A; This is a good question because it will avail me the opportunity to clear up some confusion women over fifty have about intermittent fasting. The point is, you are free to eat whatever you want during the 8-hour window period. You can think of it as fasting and a feeding window. You are not limited to three meal patterns or some arbitrary number of eating times. During this period, you can eat whatever you like. This idea needs to be tempered with some self-awareness. Yes, you can eat whatever you like, but be conscious of what types of food you are consuming and not over indulging in your eating window. As mentioned in earlier chapters, if your goal is to lose weight, the success of achieving this goal is ultimately down to creating a calorie deficit and this cannot be achieved if you cram unhealthy meals into your eating window.

Q: How long should I fast for when I start?

A: The flexibility of IF is one of the best things about it. Do not feel bad about starting with a ratio of 14:10 or 16:8. You can always adjust and progress from month to month or week to week! The key thing is to get started. Then add in resistance by shortening your eating window.

Q: Can I drink tea or coffee while I am in my fasting period?

A: Yes, you can! Remember, your fasting period is to enable your body to consume zero calories. You are free to drink water and zero calorie beverages. The reason next to zero calories need to be consumed is to avoid a change in your metabolic rate that would effectively break your fast. Black coffee and tea with no milk provide next to zero calories and would be ok to consume while fasting. However, drink it in moderation, water should be the priority. Bottled iced tea is a big no no, huge amounts of sugar are in ice tea and would definitely break your fast.

Questions About Metabolism

Q; Will Intermittent Fasting Slow Down My Metabolism?

A; Absolutely not. Studies have shown that short bursts of fasting actually boosts metabolism. However, fasting done for a more extended period, like three or more days, can reduce metabolism.

Q; Why do women over 50 have a slower metabolism?

A; As you reach fifty, you tend to reduce your regular activity and burn fewer calories. This will lead to weight gain. Age fifty and above is an age when women lose lean muscle mass, which can slow their metabolism.

Q; To lose weight, do I have to eat half as much? If not, how many calories per day are acceptable?

A: At age fifty, you need 200 fewer calories a day than you did when you were a bit younger. When you turn sixty, you will need 400-500 calories less daily. If you are moderately active before age fifty, you will need 2,000 calories per day. After fifty, it will reduce to 1,800 calories. This is a good marker to measure how many calories you eat in your feasting window. As long as your calories are below this threshold, you are giving yourself the best chance to lose that stubborn weight.

Question About Concerns and Adjustments

Q: I shouldn't have much trouble skipping breakfast during the week, but I'm worried that I can't stick to intermittent fasting on the weekends. Is that alright?

A; Absolutely. This is a good question. A good lesson for any new habit or behavior change that you want to make in your life. Just because you can't do intermittent fasting on Saturday and Sunday doesn't mean you can't do it during the week. Two days of non-fasting can't eliminate the benefits you get from doing it for the other five days.

In sum, there are many questions that women regularly ask about the reliability of intermittent fasting. Most of those questions can be best directed to your primary health provider or a nutritionist with knowledge of diet. You may need to seek professional advice or answer because you need to be guided. More so, as a woman above fifty, you may have some questions that are peculiar to you and are best resolved with your physician.

Conclusion

Reading this book should have provided answers to numerous mind-boggling questions you had on the concept of intermittent fasting. No doubt, most of your questions stemmed from finding an easier, faster, and healthier option to weight loss, considering your gender and age. It is not something new that women at your age have slowed metabolism. Notwithstanding, you have discovered the best way to lose weight and improve your metabolism without putting your health in harm's way.

Also, you have learned about different changes that would occur when your body is adapting to this new way of eating. That understanding is crucially important in helping make an informed decision about your health.

Having gone through the nitty-gritty of dieting, particularly on numerous advantages accrued to it, you can now choose one of many effective protocols that you think is the best fit for you. Remember, seeking professional help and support places you on the safe side.

More so, reading this book has opened your understanding to common mistakes that women above fifty do make when they are adopting any of the protocols. Therefore, you are advised to take note of these mistakes and the adverse effects of each of the protocols you might likely choose.

With intermittent fasting, your goal of losing weight healthily, using the best alternative is a guarantee. All you need is to adopt a protocol and ensure you stick to it until you have fully adjusted to it and achieve your health goals. Good luck!

Citations

https://www.nextavenue.org/body-changes-50-control/

https://www.ncbi.nlm.nih.gov/pmc/articles/PMC4960941/

https://www.webmd.com/healthy-aging/what-to-know-about-intermittent-fasting-for-women-after-50#2

https://jamesclear.com/the-beginners-guide-to-intermittent-fasting

https://www.healthline.com/nutrition/intermittent-fasting-guide#benefits

https://www.webmd.com/fitness-exercise/ss/slideshow-exercise-after-age-50

https://www.dietdoctor.com/keto-intermittent-fasting-completely-blown-away-changes

https://drbeckyfitness.com/intermittent-fasting-for-women-over-50/

https://www.healthline.com/nutrition/intermittent-fasting-side-effects#Who-should-avoid-intermittent-fasting?

https://www.healthline.com/nutrition/11-myths-fasting-and-meal-frequency#TOC_TITLE_HDR_11

https://www.healthline.com/nutrition/6-ways-to-do-intermittent-fasting

https://www.coachmag.co.uk/diet-plans/7206/the-pros-and-cons-of-the-168-diet

https://www.verywellfit.com/5-2-diet-pros-cons-and-how-it-works-4770014

https://www.healthline.com/nutrition/eat-stop-eat-review

https://www.healthline.com/nutrition/alternate-day-fasting-guide

https://www.medicalnewstoday.com/articles/warrior-diet

https://www.medicalnewstoday.com/articles/322293

https://www.webmd.com/healthy-aging/what-to-know-about-intermittent-fasting-for-women-after-50

https://primewomen.com/health/nutrition/benefits-of-intermittent-fasting-for-women-over-50/

https://www.womenshealthmag.com/weight-loss/a32223696/intermittent-fasting-plateau/

https://www.jns-journal.com/article/0022-510X(88)90132-3/pdf

https://www.healthline.com/nutrition/intermittent-fasting-and-weight-loss

https://www.healthline.com/nutrition/weight-loss-vs-fat-loss

https://www.verywellfit.com/how-to-take-your-body-measurements-1231126

https://www.verywellfit.com/weight-loss-and-fitness-track-progress-chart-1231119

https://healthyeating.sfgate.com/normal-weight-lose-per-week-women-10061.html

https://www.healthline.com/nutrition/10-best-weight-loss-apps

https://www.smartsheet.com/blog/essential-guide-writing-smart-goals

https://www.healthline.com/health/type-2-diabetes/intermittent-fasting-and-diabetes-safe

https://www.ncbi.nlm.nih.gov/pmc/articles/PMC6194375/

https://core.ac.uk/reader/196576423?utm_source=linkout

https://www.verywellhealth.com/diabetes-and-intermittent-fasting-4844452

https://observer.com/2017/06/most-common-intermittent-fasting-mistakes/

https://simple.life/blog/intermittent-fast-without-being-hungry/

https://lean-squad.com/blog/curb-hunger-if/

https://lean-squad.com/blog/curb-hunger-if/

https://www.sundayrest.com/blogs/sunday/how-to-sleep-well-during-fasting

https://onlinedoctor.lloydspharmacy.com/uk/lifestyle-advice/10-healthy-alternatives-to-unhealthy-food

https://www.cooksmarts.com/articles/15-healthy-alternatives-to-junk-food/

https://www.mindbodygreen.com/articles/should-you-intermittent-fast-during-menopause-hormone-expert-explains

https://lifesum.com/nutrition-explained/is-intermittent-fasting-more-important-than-calorie-counting

https://www.livestrong.com/article/74165-recommended-caloric-intake-weight-loss/

https://lifesum.com/nutrition-explained/is-intermittent-fasting-more-important-than-calorie-counting

https://lifesum.com/nutrition-explained/is-intermittent-fasting-more-important-than-calorie-counting

https://www.healthline.com/nutrition/what-breaks-a-fast

https://gwrymca.org/blog/best-exercises-women-over-50

https://www.nutrex.com/blog/pros-and-cons-of-fasted-cardio/

https://www.phillyvoice.com/pros-and-cons-working-out-empty-stomach-059991/

https://www.healthline.com/nutrition/exercise-after-eating

https://www.verywellfit.com/must-do-strength-training-women-over-50-3498202

https://www.womenshealthmag.com/uk/fitness/workouts/a31908597/workouts-for-over-50s/

https://www.fortunebusinessinsights.com/industry-reports/botulinum-toxin-market-100996

https://food.allwomenstalk.com/energizing-meals-thatll-give-you-the-boost-you-need/

https://www.cookinglight.com/eating-smart/nutrition-101/foods-diabetics-should-eat

https://www.healthline.com/nutrition/healthy-late-night-snacks

https://www.cookinglight.com/food/top-rated-recipes/best-superfast-weeknight-dinners

https://www.eatingwell.com/recipes/18055/health-condition/high-blood-pressure/

https://www.eatthis.com/collagen-recipes/

https://www.flavcity.com/5-easy-healthy-meal-prep-recipes/

https://mindovermunch.com/blog/foods-for-bone-health/

https://www.healthline.com/nutrition/11-brain-foods

https://primewomen.com/health/nutrition/fight-inflammation-with-food-not-drugs/

https://recipes.net/articles/healthy-recipes-for-low-cholesterol-diet/

https://www.healthline.com/nutrition/how-to-drink-more-water

https://miraclenoodle.com/blogs/miraclenoodle-blog/are-electrolyte-supplements-necessary-for-intermittent-fasting

https://www.span.health/blog/guide-to-electrolytes

https://www.aplaceformom.com/caregiver-resources/articles/healthy-sugar-alternatives

https://www.self.com/gallery/weight-loss-smoothies-nutritionists-swear-by

https://superfastdiet.com/20-fast-day-snack-ideas-under-100-calories-each/

https://www.healthline.com/nutrition/healthy-high-protein-snacks

https://www.womenshealthmag.com/weight-loss/a30658778/intermittent-fasting-meal-plan-men-s-health/

https://www.womenshealthmag.com/weight-loss/a30658778/intermittent-fasting-meal-plan-men-s-health/

https://www.everydayhealth.com/ketogenic-diet/intermittent-fasting-keto-how-it-works-benefits-risks-more/

https://www.bbcgoodfood.com/recipes/collection/ketogenic-diet-recipes

https://jamesclear.com/reader-mailbag-intermittent-fasting

https://www.healthline.com/nutrition/intermittent-fasting-guide

https://academic.oup.com/ehjopen/article/1/2/oeab026/6363797

https://www.nutri-align.com/fasting-electrolytes/

https://www.ncbi.nlm.nih.gov/books/NBK218740/

https://adapted-nutrition.com/blogs/news/can-you-take-electrolytes-while-intermittent-fasting

https://www.bupa.co.uk/newsroom/ourviews/ten-water-rich-foods-hydration

https://health.gov/sites/default/files/2019-09/2015-2020_Dietary_Guidelines.pdf

https://www.usda.gov/

https://www.sciencedirect.com/science/article/abs/pii/S0958694618301900

https://adapted-nutrition.com/blogs/news/can-you-take-electrolytes-while-intermittent-fasting

https://www.medicalnewstoday.com/articles/electrolytes-drinks#recommended-amount

https://www.fda.gov/food/nutrition-education-resources-materials/sodium-your-diet

https://www.nutri-align.com/fasting-electrolytes/

https://www.ncbi.nlm.nih.gov/books/NBK218740/

https://www.webmd.com/diet/foods-high-in-electrolytes

https://www.webmd.com/dan-brennan

https://healthyeating.sfgate.com/much-zinc-adult-female-8680.html

https://www.bupa.co.uk/newsroom/ourviews/ten-water-rich-foods-hydration

https://teens.webmd.com/all-about-food-labels

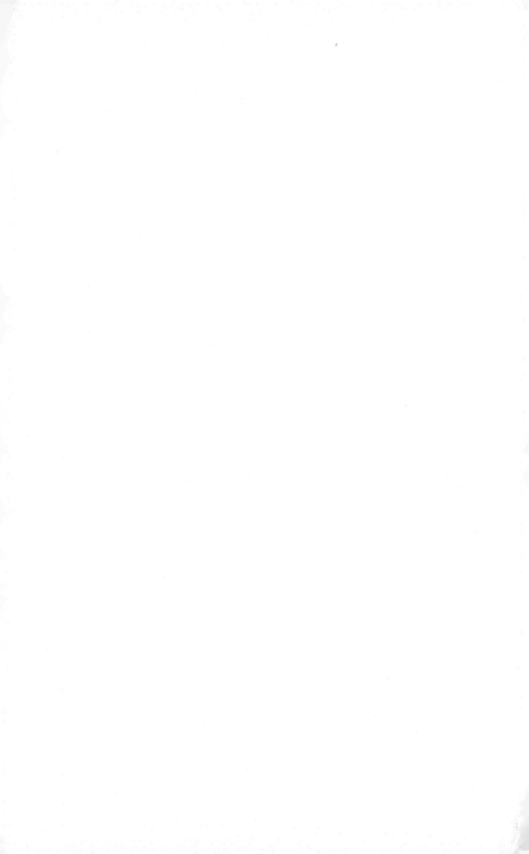

Printed in Great Britain
by Amazon

80168771R00092